MIDWIFERY

THE BASICS

Midwifery: The Basics provides an engaging and authentic insight into the midwife's world. It explores the role of the midwife as a clinician and professional, showing how midwives can support women both to achieve a healthy full-term pregnancy and a smooth transition to motherhood.

This book begins with a discussion of the context of birth and parenthood, placing midwifery in its broader social context. Topics covered include:

- the midwife as an autonomous professional;
- becoming a midwife;
- pre-conceptual and antenatal care;
- intrapartum care;
- postnatal care; and
- the specialist midwife.

Midwifery: The Basics uses the voices of mothers, fathers and midwives to illustrate the complex world of becoming, being and supporting parents. This is an essential introduction for students at undergraduate and A-Level who are approaching midwifery for the first time.

Helen Baston is Consultant Midwife in Public Health, Baby Friendly Guardian and Professional Midwifery Advocate at Sheffield Teaching Hospitals NHS Foundation Trust, UK.

The Basics

The Basics is a highly successful series of accessible guidebooks which provide an overview of the fundamental principles of a subject area in a jargon-free and undaunting format.

Intended for students approaching a subject for the first time, the books both introduce the essentials of a subject and provide an ideal springboard for further study. With over 50 titles spanning subjects from artificial intelligence (AI) to women's studies, *The Basics* are an ideal starting point for students seeking to understand a subject area.

Each text comes with recommendations for further study and gradually introduces the complexities and nuances within a subject.

For a full list of titles in this series, please visit www.routledge.com/The-Basics/book-series/B

MIDWIFERY

THE BASICS

Helen Baston

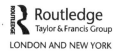

Routledge
Taylor & Francis Group

LONDON AND NEW YORK

First published 2021
by Routledge
2 Park Square, Milton Park, Abingdon, Oxon OX14 4RN

and by Routledge
52 Vanderbilt Avenue, New York, NY 10017

Routledge is an imprint of the Taylor & Francis Group, an informa business

British Library Cataloguing-in-Publication Data
A catalogue record for this book is available from the British Library

Library of Congress Cataloging-in-Publication Data
Names: Baston, Helen, 1962- author.
Title: Midwifery : the basics / Helen Baston.
Other titles: Basics (Routledge (Firm))
Description: Abingdon, Oxon ; New York, NY : Routledge, 2020. |
Series: The basics | Includes bibliographical references and index.
Identifiers: LCCN 2019058526 (print) | LCCN 2019058527 (ebook) |
ISBN 9780367146191 (hardback) | ISBN 9780367146269 (paperback) |
ISBN 9780429052750 (ebook)
Subjects: MESH: Midwifery--methods | Prenatal Care | Postnatal Care |
Nurse Midwives
Classification: LCC RG950 (print) | LCC RG950 (ebook) | NLM WQ 160 |
DDC 618.2--dc23
LC record available at https://lccn.loc.gov/2019058526
LC ebook record available at https://lccn.loc.gov/2019058527

ISBN: 978-0-367-14619-1 (hbk)
ISBN: 978-0-367-14626-9 (pbk)
ISBN: 978-0-429-05275-0 (ebk)

Typeset in Bembo
by Taylor & Francis Books

For Jo and Mary

CONTENTS

FIGURES

PREFACE

This work will draw on primary research exploring women's expectations and experiences of childbirth. It provides insight into how women perceive their caregivers during labour and, in particular, when labour ends in caesarean birth. For simplicity, the study will be referred to as the PINK study throughout this text, because the cover of the women's questionnaire was bright pink.

It examined how women felt three years after their experience and what factors influenced these emotions. It also explored how women felt looking back at their experience in relation to how they felt six weeks after the birth. In particular, issues relating to perceptions of care and carer were highlighted giving particular insights into how the way that maternity care is provided can impact on women's long-term evaluation.

For a more detailed synopsis of this research, see Appendix 1, which also has the link for the full thesis.

For convenience, the feminine third-person pronoun will be used when referring to the midwife, the masculine third-person pronoun when referring to the baby. The author recognises the valuable contribution that men also make to midwifery and this usage does not reflect any bias on her part.

Royalties from this book will be donated to UNICEF.

NOTE

This book was conceived and born before the Covid-19 pandemic was declared. However the final proofs were received and reviewed mid-crisis, enabling the addition of this note. The principles, ethos and integrity of midwifery remain the same as midwives across the world seek to support and protect women and future new families. Inevitably, there will be adaptations to the way that some aspects of care is provided. These will be developed and evaluated with women at the centre to continue to strive to achieve the core aim of being 'with woman'.

ACKNOWLEDGEMENTS

Many people have contributed directly to this book, both mid-wives and parents. This is with a view to painting a realistic picture of what it feels to be a midwife, in a range of roles and global settings. I am so grateful for all contributions, which these very busy people have kindly taken the time to produce; to reflect on and write about what midwifery means to them in their current role. They include: Adele Stanley, Alison Brodrick, Betty De Vries, Gill Walton, Hazel Walton, Sue Cooper, Sally Freeman, Marlies Rijnders, Mary Renfrew, Natalia Salim, Stephen Swan, Paula Schofield, Prue Tierney.

I also pay tribute to all the women who contributed to the PINK study, either through their questionnaire or during face-to-face interviews. Their voices have illustrated what it feels like to be a woman receiving midwifery care. I want to say a huge thank you to professors Josephine Green and Mary Renfrew, my amazing PhD supervisors whose support and wisdom facilitated the delivery of the PINK study, from which the many key quotes and insights from childbearing women are drawn and distributed throughout this book. The PINK study was funded by an award from the Health Foundation's Nursing & Allied Health Professional Research Training Fellowship Programme.

My sincere thanks also to Grace McInnes, Senior Editor at Routledge, for her warm words, patience and interest in this work and also the team of production staff who supported the transition of the manuscript into a coherent book.

Less directly, but very importantly, I would like to thank my long-suffering husband, Simon, who has listened to me deliberate over what bit should go where and read my final drafts. He has sustained me with his fantastic cooking, without which I would fade away. Our grown-up children have also put up with my absence as I have had to endure theirs. My family all know that, despite the moans and groans when there is a deadline looming, I actually do love writing, so thanks to all for your part in helping this book come to fruition.

THE CONTEXT OF BIRTH

INTRODUCTION

Each woman is unique and brings with her a background of influential health and social factors that will play a significant role in her expectations and experiences of pregnancy, birth and motherhood.

This chapter is about the social, epidemiological and emotional context of having a baby and becoming a parent to provide a backdrop for subsequent chapters which focus on midwifery and maternity care delivery. We need to understand what it means to become a mother, what impacts on women's experiences and how that appraisal might be enhanced by the care midwives give.

Before we explore the wider context of birth we must first understand the basis of all human needs – safety. There will be no context if there is no survival. Crucial to survival during childbirth is an understanding of how new life is formed and develops, how the mother's body adapts during pregnancy to protect and grow her baby. Then, through the extraordinary process of labour and birth, the baby emerges into the outside world and the mother's body makes its rapid return to its pre-pregnancy state, so it can continue its reproductive function. Her body also prepares to nurture her baby through the initiation of lactation, a process during which the mother–infant dyad is reunited.

Maslow's hierarchy of needs (1943) provides a useful model for thinking about the context of birth; it illustrates that as humans we first have basic **physiological** needs which need to be addressed above all others. Then we need to be **safe**; have nourishment, good health and a place to live. **Love** and belonging come next illustrating our need to make connections with people; family, friends and community. Only when these requirements are in place can we develop **self-esteem**, feeling good about ourselves and being recognised as individuals with respect and dignity by others. The cherry on the cake is reaching **self-actualisation**; becoming the most that we can be. This linear model does not of course capture what is now better understood, that our social connections and well-being can impact on our physical health (Holt-Lunstad et al. 2017), but that's another story.

PHYSIOLOGY

CONCEPTION AND FETAL DEVELOPMENT

Each month of the menstrual cycle an egg is released from the ovary into the fallopian tube. Following sexual intercourse, sperm migrate from the vagina, through the cervix into the uterus and swim up the fallopian tubes. When one sperm penetrates the egg, the gametes unite, and the egg is fertilised and becomes a solid ball of rapidly dividing cells (morula) and continues down the fallopian tube into the uterus where it embeds. It is called a blastocyst when it becomes a hollow ball of cells which is one-cell thick, except in one area which is thicker. The cells nearest the lumen of the blastocyst become the embryo and those nearer the outer wall, the trophoblast, become the placenta. The trophoblast further differentiates into an outer membrane known as the chorion, which surrounds the blastocyst, and an inner membrane known as the amnion, which develops into the amniotic sac. The sac begins to fill with amniotic fluid which the developing embryo floats in. The developing placenta starts to produce a hormone called human chorionic gonadotrophin (hCG) which acts on the ovaries preventing further ovulation and stimulating the production of oestrogen and progesterone and maintenance of the corpus luteum. Oestrogen and progesterone are also produced from the developing placenta and levels are adequate by 5–6 weeks, from which time production from the corpus decreases.

The organs begin to form by three weeks and with the exception of the spinal cord and brain, are completely formed by

10 weeks conceptual age. Eight weeks after fertilisation the embryo is called fetus until birth. Fetal development is incredibly rapid. By 16 weeks of pregnancy the fetus can hear, swallow, make urine and flex its arms and legs. By 20 weeks it can suck, sleep and wake, has fingernails and in female fetuses its ovaries contain eggs. By 24 weeks it has tear ducts and fingerprints and by 28 weeks it can respond to sound and open and close its eyes (ACOG 2018).

PRETERM BIRTH

Babies born before 37 completed weeks of pregnancy are defined as 'preterm'; however, many babies are born much earlier than that. Advances in nursing and medical technologies mean that many more babies are surviving than would have previously, although some are likely to have long-term health challenges or significant disability. In the UK, 10 per cent of babies survive from 22-week gestation; 60 per cent at 24 weeks; 89 per cent at 27 weeks; 95 per cent at 31 weeks; and after 34 weeks this is equivalent to full term (Tommy's 2019).

PREGNANCY

During pregnancy the female body undergoes significant changes to many organs and systems.

Progesterone, responsible for the development of the lining of the womb in preparation for implantation, continues to exert a role in preventing rejection of the embryo by suppressing contractions of the uterus. This function is taken over by the placenta and levels increase throughout pregnancy. Progesterone is responsible for breast tenderness and nausea in pregnancy, often experienced as early signs of pregnancy. It is also responsible for the growth of the uterus from its non-pregnant pear size to being able to carry a fully grown fetus. By 12 weeks of pregnancy the uterus can be palpated above the symphysis pubis, at the umbilicus at 20–22 weeks and just under the xiphisternum at 36 weeks (see Chapter 5).

GASTROINTESTINAL CHANGES

Many women experience nausea and vomiting in early pregnancy although for some it can persist throughout. In rare circumstances it can be debilitating (hyperemesis) and require intravenous fluid replacement to correct the subsequent electrolyte imbalance. It can also be associated with increased salivation (ptyalism). The gums can become swollen and bleed more readily in pregnancy. Some women experience cravings for non-foods during pregnancy, which is known as pica, but it is not known to be harmful. Oestrogen causes the appetite to be suppressed; however, progesterone stimulates it and thirst is increased; the shift in balance leads to an increased appetite in about 50 per cent of women (Coad 2011). Women often find their dietary intake increases, but there is no additional need for calories until the third trimester, and then only 300 kcal per day (NICE 2008a).

Progesterone's impact on smooth muscle tone means that the tone of the oesophageal sphincter is relaxed and acid from the stomach causes an unpleasant burning sensation or heartburn. The intestine and colon also become more relaxed and motility is reduced, leading to an increased risk of constipation.

CARDIOVASCULAR CHANGES

During early pregnancy the blood pressure falls slightly, which can lead some women to feel faint. Then the blood volume starts to increase by as much as 30–50 per cent, which is accommodated by an increased number of blood vessels, stimulated by oestrogen, and relaxation of the smooth muscle of the vessel wall, caused by progesterone. The overall impact on the cardiovascular system gives rise to an increased cardiac output, as a result of increased heart rate and stroke volume of the slightly enlarged heart. Blood pressure (diastolic) is lower in the first two-thirds of pregnancy and returns to its pre-pregnancy value by the end of pregnancy.

It is usual for most women to experience some swelling (oedema) in their hands, feet and ankles due to the effects of reduced venous return because of the space occupied by the uterus and the increased laxity of the blood vessels. The increased blood volume is not accompanied by a corresponding increase in plasma protein or red cells hence fluid is more likely to leak from the capillaries into the tissues. Elevation of the legs while sitting can help reduce the swelling, as can moderate exercise, such as brisk walking and swimming (PHE 2019a).

The blood red cell mass only increases by up to 20 per cent, from about 12 weeks of pregnancy. To meet the requirements for iron in pregnancy, the woman needs to have good iron stores pre-conceptually, despite increased iron absorption during pregnancy. Routine supplementation with iron is therefore recommended in countries where the diet of the population is poor (WHO 2017a); it is not currently recommended in the UK (NICE 2008b).

Pregnancy is a time when the risk of thrombosis is increased because there is venous stasis, increased fibrin and reduced fibrinolytic activity and endothelial damage (Devis & Knuttinen 2017). It is thought that this is an evolutionary development to protect women from haemorrhage during the birth. However, thrombosis is the leading cause of maternal death in England (Knight et al. 2018); a risk that increases with maternal age and body mass index.

RENAL CHANGES

The anatomy of the kidneys changes during pregnancy because of the impact of progesterone, which causes the ureters to lose tone and become elongated. Urinary stasis is increased and can lead to urinary tract infection (UTI). There is increased glomerular filtration and tubular reabsorption, leading to increased sodium and subsequent fluid retention. The bladder is under pressure from the growing uterus in the first trimester, until the uterus becomes an abdominal organ, leading to increased frequency of micturition. When the fetal head (96 per cent of babies present head-first at term) starts to engage in the pelvis towards the end of pregnancy, these symptoms return.

RESPIRATORY CHANGES

To increase the efficiency of gaseous exchange tidal volume increases and alveolar ventilation increases due to the relaxation of smooth muscle in the bronchioles. Also, the softening of cartilage and muscle in the thorax facilitates chest expansion. Some women become breathless in pregnancy and anaemia or heart anomaly should be ruled out before this is attributed to reduced space below the diaphragm. Oedema of the vocal cords can lead to a deepening of the voice.

SKELETAL CHANGES

Due to the impact of the hormones progesterone and relaxin on the joints, the symphysis pubis can become more mobile and even separate. The sacroiliac joints in the pelvis also become more flexible to increase the pelvic outlet for birth. Combined with the above and the increased weight of the gravid uterus and breasts, pregnant women can appear to waddle and arch their backs when they walk.

LABOUR AND BIRTH

The mystique of pregnancy and childbirth continues as we still have a lot to learn about the complex interplay of the factors which lead to the onset of spontaneous labour. Whilst it is thought that fetal factors have a role to play when labour starts, the mechanisms are unclear.

The cervix is the gatekeeper, holding the fetus in the uterus. For the baby to be born, the cervix needs to become fully dilated to enable the baby to pass from the uterus, through the vagina and to the outside world. In obstetric terms the dilatation of the cervix is measured from closed (0 cm) to fully open (10 cm) and this is usually assessed by regular vaginal examinations. During pregnancy, the cervix of the primigravid woman is closed and has thickness, somewhat like a doughnut with a closed hole in shape. Towards the end of pregnancy, the woman will experience 'Braxton-Hicks' contractions, which are usually painless uterine contractions. These herald the beginning of the long process of softening and preparing the cervix for dilatation, but they may be experienced for several weeks before labour starts.

LATENT PHASE

This is the pre-labour phase, which is variable between individuals. It can start with what are experienced as regular, painful contractions which may last a few hours and then fade away. Other women experience mild, irregular contractions before getting into a more established pattern. During this time the cervix begins to soften and dilate up to 4 cm.

During the latent phase and with uterine contractions the length of the cervix shortens, which is known as 'effacement'. The uterus and the cervix are continuous with each other. As the cervix effaces and softens its thickness becomes taken up into the body of the uterus, from the external cervical os upwards. In women who have previously given birth, effacement and dilatation can occur simultaneously.

Due to the unique property of the myometrial muscle fibres, following contraction, they become shorter and retract. The top (fundus) of the uterus becomes thicker and during a contraction, pressure is exerted in line with the long axis of the baby. The lower segment of the uterus thins and accommodates the head of the baby as it descends. Pressure of a well-fitting fetal head on the cervix gives rise to the release of local prostaglandins, which in turn stimulates the release of oxytocin which causes the uterus to contract. Uterine contractions in turn assist with the application of the pressure of the presenting part on the cervix and so this cycle is self-perpetuating. However, if the head is not fitting well, perhaps because the baby is in an awkward position or a full bladder or bowel are causing the head to be high in the pelvis, then uterine contractions will be less efficient. Whilst the bag of waters surrounding the baby remain intact, they form forewaters in front of the baby's head which enables the pressure to be distributed evenly over the cervix. This bag of amniotic fluid can 'break' at any time, before or during any stage of labour, and whilst often portrayed in the media as a dramatic gush leaving the woman standing in a puddle, it is often a much more subtle leak.

FIRST STAGE OF LABOUR

During this active stage of labour, dilation of the cervix, from 4 to 10 cm, begins to accelerate at a rate of approximately 1–2 cm per hour depending on parity. Contractions are now lasting longer (30–60 seconds), closer together and more painful. During this stage the baby continues to be active. The mother is encouraged to engage her coping strategies, such as breathing techniques, the use of water, movement and music to help her cope with the powerful contractions (see Chapter 6). Her cardiac output increases due to increasing circulating blood volume and venous return. She produces increased adrenaline in response to the pain and stress of labour which can impact on placental blood flow to the fetus; it is therefore important that she is supported to relax and breathe gently between contractions.

SECOND STAGE OF LABOUR

This is defined as from full dilatation to the birth of the baby. The birth of the baby is facilitated by the expulsive forces of the uterus and the muscles of the diaphragm accompanied by the involuntary bearing down efforts of the mother. The soft tissue resistance of the vagina and pelvic floor yield to the descent and progress of the baby through the birth canal. With each contraction the fetus advances and then recedes; the uterine muscle retracts and the fundus continues to thicken, helping the fetus to advance. There reaches a point where the widest part of the head (the biparietal diameter) passes through the pelvis and 'crowning' occurs. The perineum stretches and, with encouragement, the woman is supported to breathe the head out. The head is usually born with the next contraction negotiating the curve of the pelvis. The head then turns (restitution) as the shoulders engage with the pelvic floor and rotate; the shoulders are born with the next contraction and the baby is passed to its mother, cord intact.

THIRD STAGE OF LABOUR

Following the birth of the baby, the uterus contracts and the placenta separates from the uterine wall aided by the formation of a retro-placental clot. The muscle fibres of the myometrium tighten around the exposed maternal blood vessels to form 'living ligatures' (Coad 2011). Depending on the method of management of the third stage requested by the mother (see Chapter 6) the mother will either push the placenta out or its delivery will be assisted by controlled cord traction.

THE PHYSIOLOGY OF THE PUERPERIUM

Following the expulsion of the placenta and for the next six weeks is the postnatal period, also known as the puerperium. During this time the woman's reproductive system body returns to its near pre-

pregnancy state, give or take some stretch marks, scars and excess weight. The length of time her body takes to recover will depend on her mode of birth, pre-pregnancy fitness, age and parity.

HORMONES

Once the placenta has separated, the levels of hormones it produced (progesterone and oestrogen) begin to fall and are reduced to pre-pregnancy levels within 72 hours. Levels of follicle-stimulating hormone (FSH) begin to increase and are usually at pre-pregnancy levels by about three weeks thus preparing her body for future fertility. However, the levels of luteinising hormone (LH), required to stimulate ovulation, will depend on whether a woman is breastfeeding and how often. Prolactin, produced during breastfeeding, plays an important role in suppressing ovulation.

CONTRACTION OF THE UTERUS

Immediately after completion of the third stage of labour, the uterus is firm and well contracted. It can be palpated by the midwife externally at about the level of the umbilicus, or just below, and feels like a cricket ball. The hormone oxytocin is released from the posterior pituitary gland leading to intermittent contractions of the myometrium, which helps maintain sustained uterine contraction.

It is vital, literally, that this process occurs efficiently, otherwise there is the potential for maternal haemorrhage from the placental site. The myometrial muscle fibres contract around the exposed blood vessels and they become occluded. Also, with this uterine contraction, the uterine walls are pressed against each other which further reduces blood loss. Blood clotting mechanisms are activated and thus bleeding from the placental site is further minimised. There is potential for any of these aspects to be compromised if, for example, fragments of placenta or membranes are retained within the uterine cavity or if a blood clotting abnormality has developed.

INVOLUTION OF THE UTERUS

Immediately after the birth, the post-gravid uterus weighs about 900 g. Over the next few days and weeks, its mass reduces and approximately

50 per cent is lost in the next seven days. By the end of the puerperium it will be back to its pre-pregnancy weight of about 60 g. This happens due to the combined processes of 'autolysis' or 'self-digestion' brought about by the release of enzymes from the myometrial cells, the cells from the lining of the occluded blood vessels and macrophages. The myometrial cells become smaller and the bulk of the uterus is reduced. By about ten days postnatally the uterus can no longer be palpated abdominally, although this involution is slower in women who have had a caesarean section.

LOCHIA

The blood loss following childbirth is called lochia and changes over time. For about the first three days the red loss contains blood and decidua from the placental site. The volume reduces and becomes pink or brown in colour containing decidua and epithelial cells from the vagina as well as leucocytes and mucus. Some white/yellow discharge may persist for up to six weeks which contains leucocytes, cervical mucous and serous fluid. Lochia should not contain blood clots or smell offensive; both are signs of a potential infection.

THE CERVIX

The entrance to the uterus reforms quickly after childbirth and after one week it is almost closed, although it never returns to its pre-pregnancy shape and the external cervical os becomes slit shaped.

VAGINA

The rugae or ridges of the vagina disappear during a vaginal birth. After about three weeks, the vagina becomes shorter and the rugae begin to return, returning to pre-pregnancy size by six weeks. The rugae become less pronounced with repeated childbirth.

PERINEUM

The body of skin and muscle between the entrance to the vagina and the anus undergoes considerable stretching and displacement during vaginal childbirth. It is common for some trauma to be sustained and this can be superficial such as grazing or involve significant muscle damage. Where the skin and/or muscle is not aligned, surgical repair by the midwife may be needed. Where there is extensive damage, involving the anal sphincter, surgical repair by an obstetrician in theatre will be required. The perineum has an excellent blood supply and usually heals quickly. Pelvic floor exercises will assist with the restoration in muscle tone and help prevent urinary and faecal incontinence.

THE PHYSIOLOGY OF BREASTFEEDING

Breastfeeding and the production of breastmilk is a complex combination of amazing physiology and maternal resilience. Essentially what is needed for successful breastfeeding is a combination of close and sustained mother–infant contact, effective positioning and attachment at the breast and feeding whenever the baby or mother want.

During pregnancy the breast tissue begins to change due to the effect of oestrogen, which supports the development of the ducts, and progesterone, which supports the development of the glandular tissue. Levels of prolactin increase throughout pregnancy, stimulating growth and differentiation of the breast tissue, but milk production is inhibited by placental hormone progesterone. Once the baby is born, however, and the placenta expelled, there is a drop in the levels of progesterone and oestrogen.

The importance of skin-to-skin contact, especially in the first hour after birth, cannot be overemphasised. Oxytocin levels are running high and the mother is ideally placed and programmed to tune into her baby at this time. If placed in direct skin contact with its mother the baby can make its own way to the breast (Brimdyr et al. 2017). Covered in a warm dry towel and supported by its mother the baby is alert and relaxed. About three minutes after birth it starts to move, open its eyes and move its head. Then it begins to make rooting and mouthing movements. It may rest a while before crawling to the breast with short bursts of activity. After about 45 minutes it familiarises itself with the mother's nipple, touching and licking, putting its hand in its mouth before eventually attaching to the nipple and feeding. Most babies usually fall asleep about 90 minutes after the birth, therefore it is important that this process is not interrupted as the baby must then start back at the beginning and may fall asleep before it reaches its goal.

When the baby suckles, prolactin, produced in the anterior pituitary gland, is released into the bloodstream and acts on the alveoli in the breast to stimulate milk production. Prolactin levels begin to rise after 10 minutes and are highest after about 30 minutes of starting to feed, to support milk production for the next feed. Levels are especially high at night and the more the baby sucks the more milk is produced. Prolactin is particularly important for the establishment of the milk supply in the early weeks.

The other essential hormone in the process of breastfeeding is oxytocin. This is also produced when the baby sucks or if the mother sees or thinks about her baby. It is made in the hypothalamus and stored in the posterior pituitary gland and released into the bloodstream, acting on the myoepithelial cells that surround the alveolar sacs, the cluster of cells where milk is made. Milk then flows along the ducts to the baby. The release of oxytocin can be inhibited by emotions such as fear, pain, fatigue and separation from her baby. Therefore, the environment in which feeding takes place should enable her to feel safe and private. She should have adequate pain relief if needed and be supported in close skin-to-skin contact with her baby.

The production of milk is locally controlled, which means that if milk is not removed from the breast, either through feeding the baby or expression, then the polypeptide called 'feedback inhibitor of lactation' (FIL) builds up and milk production stops. This is also significant for successful breastfeeding because if the baby is not latched on well, there will not be efficient milk removal and FIL will build up. Similarly, if the baby does not feed well and does not stimulate the breast, prolactin levels will diminish.

MICROBIOME

There are many factors that influence our microbiome, beginning with exposure in utero and during birth. The impact of disruption to bacterial communities within the gut includes an increased risk of allergies, autoimmune disorders, obesity and diabetes (Tamburini et al. 2016). The developing fetus may be exposed to bacteria in utero, via the maternal bloodstream or ascending via the genital tract and this is known to be a factor in preterm birth.

The first milk *colostrum* is rich in many bioactive factors including antibodies and lactoferrin to prevent infection and is also a source of growth factors and anti-inflammatory agents. Produced in small quantities, it is sufficient to sustain to the baby's nutritional requirements in the first days until the mature milk supply is established. Breastmilk contains hundreds of biologically active factors that support the development of a healthy immune system and maturation of the gut, supporting healthy microbial colonisation (Ballard & Morrow 2013). If formula feeds are introduced then there are significant consequences for the establishment of feeding and for the baby's gut microbiome. O'Sullivan et al. (2015) call for more research to examine the impact of this practice, which has the potential to increase pro-inflammatory factors.

SAFETY

Having established that the processes of conception, childbirth and breastfeeding are the result of complex, evolutionary mechanisms, we must acknowledge that our modern-day meddling may have given rise to potentially challenging outcomes. Access to our basic needs for good health, to be well fed, breathe clean air, have access to green spaces and a place of sanctuary are socially and financially determined.

EPIDEMIOLOGY

To identify and examine the root causes of differences between and within populations and their subgroups, we need to have access to tools that measure health trends and differentiate the associated causal factors. The discipline of epidemiology provides this framework and is essential for public health to progress; providing evidence to inform understanding where we are now and how interventions can make a difference. Epidemiology is defined as:

> the study (scientific, systematic, and data-driven) of the distribution (frequency, pattern) and determinants (causes, risk factors) of health-related states and events (not just diseases) in specified populations

(neighbourhood, school, city, state, country, global). It is also the application of this study to the control of health problems (CDC 2006:5).

This definition clearly describes the components of this discipline and its ability to influence key health developments, including maternity services and the wider community globally. Originating from the study of the what, who, where, when and why of communicable diseases, this enquiry method has expanded to explore how behaviours and genetics have impacted on health at a population level. Modig et al. (2017:5) make a clear argument for the monitoring of disease trends in order to 'plan implementations and actions aimed at improving health and for evaluating such action'.

Monitoring and evaluating programmes designed to improve maternal and child health requires access to robust data. Systems that are often taken for granted in high-income countries, such as compulsory registration of births, are integral to effective monitoring of progress made. However, it is not only important to understand the direction of travel in terms of health improvements, but also to learn how changes were implemented, who they worked for and how they were evaluated.

SOCIAL DETERMINANTS OF HEALTH

In addition to the inequalities in provision and access to key health services across the UK and globally, there are a range of social determinants of health that also conspire to perpetuate disadvantage. These social factors are those which are found in relation to a person's income and influence that comes with their living or working conditions. For example, living in a small terraced house alongside a busy polluted main road will create health challenges not experienced by people living in a more affluent leafy green suburb. In summary, social determinants of health include: income, education, employment, stress, housing, race, disability, food, transport, social exclusion, early child development, social support, gender, etc.

The interaction of these factors is complex. For example, it may be public policy that there are Children's Centres where parents can access support services to mitigate the challenges of social isolation and poor employment opportunities. However, inadequate transport systems may not enable access to these facilities by the people who really need them; indeed, the car park may be full of the cars of women who can drive across town to take up the valuable resources they offer. Similarly, whilst there may be schools and supermarkets in all neighbourhoods, their quality and the facilities they offer are likely to be varied and inequalities of access persist. In addition, social norms will also have a part to play in the culture of a neighbourhood and what is perceived as appropriate behaviour by peers.

Marmot (2010) highlighted the huge social gradients for many health outcomes and these indicators have recently been updated (Marmot 2017). The difference in life expectancy between men in Kensington is 83 years compared with 74 years in Blackpool and for women in Kensington it is 86 years compared with 79 years in Manchester. There are also inequality gradients within local authorities by as much as 15 years. The overall life expectancy had been increasing by one year in every five years for women but this has now slowed to one in every ten years. Indicators for children are equally concerning; for example, the proportion of children being eligible for free school meals is increasing year on year. Inevitably, the general health of the population is reflected in maternal health outcomes, which will now be described.

MATERNAL BIRTH OUTCOMES

DEMOGRAPHICS

The birth rate in England is declining; from 652,638 in 2008–9 to 603,766 in 2018–19, which is a reduction of 3.3 per cent from 2017–18 (NHS Digital 2019). Births amongst women under 20 years totalled 16,956 in 2018–19 and has more than halved since 2008–9. However, the percentage of women giving birth in the 30–39 age group has increased by 7 per cent since 2008–9. Women who are older are more likely to experience obstetric intervention; for example, the caesarean birth rate is 46 per cent for women over 40 years of age (NHS Digital 2019).

PUBLIC HEALTH

Access to early antenatal care is recommended for early access to screening and dating of the pregnancy (NICE 2008b); however, only 61 per cent had their first antenatal assessment between 8–11 weeks of pregnancy. Smoking prevalence in all populations is decreasing yet it remains high in young pregnant women; 30 per cent of under 20-year-olds compared with 6 per cent of women over 40 years. Body mass index increased with age; the proportion in the obese range (>30 BMI) was lowest for those aged under 20 years and highest (25 per cent) in women aged over 40 years. It is recommended that all women take folic acid supplements pre-conceptually to reduce the risk of having a baby with an open neural tube defect: 83 per cent of women report taking folic acid prior to or on confirmation of pregnancy (NHS Digital 2019).

TEENAGE PREGNANCY

The under 18 years' conception rate in the UK is now at its lowest level since 1969 (PHE 2018). Teenage pregnancy rates tend to be higher, however, in countries where there is no access to free contraception and where parental consent is required for termination of pregnancy (Part et al. 2013). Whilst they have declined throughout Europe, the UK under 18 years' conception rate is still comparatively high at 17.8 per 1,000 (PHE 2019b). Teenage parents are vulnerable and more likely to live in poverty, have low birth weight babies, smoke, have poor mental health and less likely to breastfeed than adult parents (PHE 2018).

MODE OF BIRTH

Whilst spontaneous birth still accounts for the majority of birth in England (57 per cent) (NHS Digital 2019), there has been a consistent rise in the proportion of babies that are born by caesarean section. Caesarean birth is often classified in two categories: 'elective' (planned) or 'emergency' (all others).

Once a rare procedure, occurring in fewer than 3 per cent of births in the 1950s, rates have risen from 19.7 per cent of births in 2000 to 26.2 per cent in 2015 (Wise 2018). In 2019, caesarean section rates in England reached the alarming rate of 30 per cent (NHS Digital 2019); 13 per cent elective and 17 per cent emergency. Twelve per cent of births were assisted by instrumentation, either ventouse or forceps. Most births have a spontaneous onset;

however, this has declined from 69 per cent in 2008–9 to 50 per cent in 2018–19, with 17 per cent being elective caesarean and 33 per cent are now induced.

Women who experience caesarean birth today do so within a culture that regards this mode of birth as a safe, sometimes preferable, alternative to vaginal birth. In the current context of intrapartum care in the UK, women who have a caesarean birth are likely to be cared for in a maternity unit with midwifery, obstetric, anaesthetic and paediatric disciplines working together to support the needs of the family unit. Women are generally healthy when they have their caesarean although some will be suffering from complications of pregnancy and/or from existing morbidity but it is generally perceived as a safe procedure.

Various strategies have been employed to reduce the escalation of caesarean section rates, including: external cephalic version (for babies who present by breech), one-to-one support in labour and facilitating vaginal birth after previous caesarean. Their success, however, depends on the prevailing cultural and social circumstances at a population level as well as the individual attitudes of the obstetricians and the women they care for.

BABIES AND BREASTFEEDING

Seven per cent of babies were born with a low birth weight of less than 2.5 kg, 1.2 per cent were less than 1.5 kg. The majority (99 per cent) of term babies were born with an Apgar score of 7 or more. Current annual breastfeeding rates at 6–8 weeks (2018–19) are 46.2 per cent, which shows an upward trend from the previous year's 43.1 per cent (NHS Digital 2019). Skin-to-skin contact at birth is well embedded in maternity care in the UK with 82 per cent of mothers who had a baby born at 37 weeks or more having skin-to-skin with an hour of birth; 75 per cent of babies received breastmilk for their first feed. Women who choose to breastfeed are more likely to come from an area of higher socioeconomic status, be more highly educated and older than women who formula feed their babies.

MATERNAL MORTALITY IN THE UK

A key measure of the health of a nation are its mortality rates, which often reflect underlying inequalities and access and uptake of services. In the UK, it is mandatory to report all maternal deaths and each one is subject to a confidential enquiry into its cause and related care factors. Each Confidential Enquiry into Maternal Death (CEMD) report covers a three-year period.

Maternal deaths are defined as deaths of women while pregnant or within 42 days of delivery, miscarriage or termination of pregnancy, from any cause related to or aggravated by the pregnancy or its management, but not from accidental or incidental causes. Maternal deaths are classified as: direct (resulting from a complication associated with pregnancy, birth or puerperium); indirect (due to previous existing disease exacerbated by pregnancy); late (direct or indirect deaths occurring between 42 days to 1 year after pregnancy); and coincidental (unrelated to the influence of pregnancy). Over the years there has been a general trend in a reduction of direct deaths compared with indirect deaths, suggesting that maternity care is now more effective and that more women are coming to pregnancy with pre-existing disease.

In the UK the leading cause of direct death up to 42 days after birth for the period 2012–14 was thrombosis and thromboembolism, followed by haemorrhage and suicide. However, suicide is the leading cause of direct death up to one year after birth. Cardiac disease is the leading cause of indirect death (Knight et al. 2018). Of particular note is that women from black ethnic backgrounds are five times more likely to die compared to white women. Death rates are also higher in older women and women from deprived areas, 57 per cent were overweight or obese and 16 per cent were known to social services and therefore known to be vulnerable. Access to maternity care was also a factor with only 26 per cent of those women who received antenatal care having booked before 10 weeks of pregnancy and attended for all the recommended visits (NICE 2008b).

The publication of this report is now annual, still covering a three-year period but without the delay in reporting the trends. This enables a timelier review of why women die; each maternity service can now review its own care pathways against the recommendations of the report. It has undoubtedly resulted in fewer maternal deaths because of changes in practice it has championed (Kee 2005).

GLOBAL MATERNAL HEALTH

As well as the variations in health that are socially determined by women globally, because of 'the circumstances in which they are born, grow, live, work and age' (WHO CSDH 2008:26) there are huge variations in maternal health across the world, reflecting inequalities regarding access to safe maternity care. The World Health Organization have developed Programme Reporting Standards (PRSs) to elicit relevant information to determine what works in sexual, reproductive, maternal, newborn, child and adolescent health (SRMNCAH) programmes (WHO 2017b).

Timely and skilled healthcare provision in pregnancy, childbirth and in the postnatal period is essential in order to prevent the catastrophic impact of infection, haemorrhage and complications that early identification could have averted. Data is collated on the percentage of births attended by 'skilled health personnel' (doctor, nurse and/or midwife) and it demonstrates that fewer than half of the births in many low- and middle-income countries (LMIC) have such attendance, compared with the majority of upper-middle and high-income countries where skilled care is provided for more than 90 per cent of women (UNICEF/WHO 2018).

GLOBAL MATERNAL MORTALITY RATES

Since the commitment made in 2000 to the eight Millennium Development Goals (MDGs) the progress towards a global reduction in Maternal Mortality Ratio (MMR) has been significant. For example, in 2000 there were 451,000 maternal deaths globally compared with 295,000 in 2017, representing a reduction of 38.4 per cent (WHO 2019:41). The MMR is presented as the number of maternal deaths per 100,000 live births and varies considerably between and within countries. Globally the MMR in 2017 was 211 (per 100,000 live births) yet 542 in sub-Saharan Africa; 157 in Southern Asia; 10 in Europe; and 7 in Australia and New Zealand (WHO 2019:41). However, taking a closer look at specific populations, some even more alarming data estimates suggest that the MMR is as high as 1,150 in South Sudan, 1,140 in Chad and 1,120 in Sierra Leone (WHO 2019:34). These rates are estimates based on the available data, which is variable in quality and quantity.

Access to a caesarean section when clinically indicated saves both mothers' and infants' lives; however, as an intervention not without consequences, its use should be used judiciously. International caesarean rates vary widely between countries, from 0.6 per cent in South Sudan to 58.9 per cent in the Dominican Republic (Boatin et al. 2018). In hospitals in Brazil, 55.6 per cent of births were by caesarean in 2015 and in China in 2016, the rate was 41.3 per cent (Boerma et al. 2018).

The World Health Organization had recommended since 1985 that a rate above 10–15 per cent is unjustified on health grounds and this continues to be widely supported (Betran et al. 2015). This statement has been reviewed and replaced by a statement that makes a more conservative recommendation of a rate no higher than 10 per cent (WHO 2015). The review also advocates the use of the Robson (2001) classification system to enable the collation of robust data to inform further reviews. However, it is argued that due to changes in the demographics of many countries, such as increasing maternal age, a rate of approximately 20 per cent is optimal (Robson & de Costa 2017). It has been suggested that rising caesarean section rates are associated with increased maternal choice, as observed in Chile (Elejalde & Giolito 2019). An increase in birth in private hospitals, and delivery by doctors rather than midwives, has also resulted in an increase in caesarean section rates.

To address the considerable concerns about global maternal mortality there needs to extensive investment and action by governments across the world. However, such work would need to be evidence based, comprehensively scoped and modelled with authority. This is exactly what a group of leading midwifery academics and statistical experts achieved in the groundbreaking *Lancet* series on midwifery.

This important series of four papers presents the case for global nations to recognise and invest in the role of the midwife. It begins with a review of four countries' attempts to improve survival rates in mothers and infants (Van Lerberghe et al. 2014). It demonstrated that to achieve this, there needed to be significant commitment and investment in the multiple dimensions of quality at a technical, interpersonal and organisational level.

The second paper is a comprehensive exploration of the scope of midwifery practice and what potential outcomes could be improved by midwifery care (Renfrew at al 2014). Using the International Confederation of Midwives definition of the midwife (ICM 2011) to elucidate the full scope of the midwife's role and a multi-method approach to identifying relevant sources of evidence, a framework for high-quality maternal and newborn care was developed. Mothers' views were sought and included, and the interventions highlighted as relevant were then examined for effectiveness. This framework can be used for planning future services where skilled midwifery care saves lives and strengthens women's own capacity to promote health.

In the third paper, the Lives Saved Tool (LiST) was used to estimate the impact of discrete midwifery interventions, by combining the evidence of the effectiveness of these interventions with their coverage and mortality rates and causes (Homer et al. 2014). It is not possible to model the other undoubted impact of midwifery interventions, such as women's perception of their experience, impact on ill health and well-being. Seventy-eight countries were included in the detailed modelling. Based on a conservative increase in midwifery coverage of 10 per cent every five years, it was estimated that there would be a 27.4 per cent reduction in maternal deaths in countries with a low Human Development Index (HDI) where the absolute numbers of deaths would be greatest based on the size of those populations. Similar reductions were also seen in the model for stillbirths and neonatal deaths. The authors considered four scenarios, comparing options where universal midwifery coverage would ultimately be achieved and also what might happen to maternal death rates if coverage was reduced. Further analysis was undertaken exploring the addition of specialist medical care, although the impact was less pronounced. They concluded that their modelling

> highlights the need for midwifery, specifically midwives, to be part of a team within a functional and enabling health system that has a skilled health workforce with the appropriate competencies and is

based in the community and hospital or health facility. This is an important step towards ensuring that women can have access to a quality midwifery service that can provide the maternal and newborn health interventions, and preventive health-care strategies (Homer et al. 2014:1153–4).

In the final paper of the series the findings of the previous three papers are summarised and the practical considerations about how the findings can be implemented are presented (Hoope-Bender et al. 2014). It was described how a whole system approach would be needed, not only to scale up the education of future midwives to meet the demand, but also in terms of regulation, clinical environments and human resource processes. How to measure midwifery productivity would also need careful consideration, to ensure that quality of care was not compromised by financial concerns. It was acknowledged that with the increased demand for services in a tight labour market, care would need to be taken to avoid the commercialisation of childbirth.

The optimism and opportunity this important series created has been laid down as a challenge for global nations to invest in the framework and take the 'opportunity to transform health, education, and social systems to make maternal, newborn, and child health a reality for all' (Hoope-Bender et al. 2014:1233).

THE SUSTAINABLE DEVELOPMENT GOALS (SDGS)

These 17 SDGs are a call to action by the United Nations General Assembly, agreed in 2015 for achievement by 2030. They built on the moderate success of the Millennium Development Goals agreed in 2000; one of which was to 'improve maternal health'.

It is recognised that for a healthy and sustainable workforce, economy and society, more needs to be done to protect the mothers who nurture future generations. Every Woman Every Child (EWEC 2015) was launched in 2010 at the MDG summit and underpins the global strategy objectives: survive, thrive and transform. Monitoring of these commitments shows that investment focuses mostly on the 'survive' element, then the 'thrive' aspect, with much to do in relation to developing services that will ultimately 'transform' the lives of future generation (PMNCH/WHO 2018).

The SDGs are ambitions set for a better world, in which poverty and hunger are conquered and the planet is saved from climate change, war and health inequalities. However, to meet these goals resources are required to address the need to create skilled roles, provide education and clean water; there is much work to do. Whilst there is no longer a specific goal focusing on maternal health, many aspects of the new programme include ambitions to address the issues childbearing women face, including: no poverty, gender equality, clean water and access to clean water (United Nations 2019).

Based on the previous rate of change in addressing maternal mortality rates, the SDG to eliminate preventable maternal deaths will not be achieved by 2030. In 2018, a declaration was made that primary healthcare is the most cost-effective way to achieve global health coverage (UNICEF/WHO 2018). There is much work to do to ensure that mothers and babies around the world are nurtured in a safe and protective midwifery embrace.

LOVE, BELONGING AND CONNECTION

Having explored some of the fundamental safety needs and the health and obstetric outcomes of childbearing women, we now move on to explore how Maslow's next tier in the hierarchy of basic human needs is experienced in the context of motherhood and midwifery.

COMPASSIONATE CARE

Often described as fundamental to good quality maternity care (Byrom & Downe 2015), compassionate care is achieved when the carer acts to relieve suffering. To do so, however, the midwife must first be able to recognise a woman's distress and be emotionally available for her. Midwives need to be able to manage their own emotions and tune into the needs of the woman. They must be aware of their demeanour and the messages that their body language is conveying; coping with uncertainty whilst maintaining a personal and optimistic approach is a key midwifery skill.

Compassionate care transcends empathy, through the behaviour and engagement of professionals with women, as the following vignette, written by a senior midwife, demonstrates:

One of the most significant truths I have uncovered over the years is that kindness is the most important quality a midwife brings to the birthing room. We can all learn how to cannulate, suture, read a CTG etc but women won't remember all that stuff, they remember you holding their hand, rubbing an achy leg and by maintaining total belief in their awesomeness.

One example was a woman came into the labour ward assessment area in a state of obvious distress. I saw her sitting and crying in the waiting room. I invited her into a room on the labour ward, not knowing if she was in labour or was even pregnant but knowing I could not leave her in that state. I just let her cry for a while, fetched her tissues, got her some water and held her hand until she wanted to talk to me. Eventually she told me the story of a previous birth which she has experienced as traumatic and she felt like she was labouring again but was terrified of it all happening again. She had had pre-eclampsia before. I reassured her I would stay with her no matter what and between us we would try our best to have a better time. As it turned out she had pre-eclampsia again. I stayed with her, I used mobile monitoring so she could walk around, played her music, did some massage and we laughed. Her partner was very funny. She had a normal birth on all fours.

She sent me a letter sometime after and said it was the kindness she experienced in those first moments that made all the difference; it made her feel safe and allowed her to believe she could have the birth she so wanted. Just kindness. Being kind isn't difficult but it really makes a difference. My last student said if she had learnt one thing from me it was that we should always be kind even if it is difficult or we don't feel like it. An important lesson to learn, I feel.

Adele Stanley, midwife, UK

The love and connection that midwives have with women and their families is a vital part of maternity care. Midwives who have helped the woman connect with her growing baby throughout pregnancy are helping her lay the foundations for a strong emotional attachment with her baby.

OXYTOCIN

Often described as the 'love hormone' oxytocin has a vital role in establishing and maintaining social connection. Childbirth guru

Sheila Kitzinger is renowned for the philosophy that the baby's place of birth should be as intimate as the room where it was conceived (Kitzinger 1983). Dimly lit, warm and comfortable birthing rooms support the release of oxytocin during labour. Oxytocin not only helps the uterus contract; it helps reduce stress, anxiety and pain and promotes friendly social interactions (Uvnäs-Moberg et al. 2019).

Oxytocin levels increase as labour progresses and there is a large pulse of oxytocin after vaginal birth (Uvnäs-Moberg et al. 2019). Skin-to-skin contact with the baby immediately after birth further supports its release into the mother's bloodstream, and supports bonding and attachment and helps reduce both maternal and new-born stress (Crenshaw 2014). It therefore makes sense that labour and birth care should enable the woman's oxytocin levels to remain high and not be disrupted by the negative impact of the hormones cortisol and adrenaline, which are released at times of fear and stress.

BABY BRAIN DEVELOPMENT

We are now aware of the importance of the early years of a child's life on its brain development and future prospects. By the time a child starts school there are already wide variations in ability between classmates. Yet these differences in cognitive development can begin early in the antenatal period, depending on parental input. The first 1,000 days of a child's life (conception to age two years) are a particularly critical period when its brain is developing and neural pathways are becoming established. It has been described as a 'unique period of opportunity' (Cusick & Georgieff 2019). The implications of early interactions may have lifetime impact on a child's ability to socialise and affiliate with others in the future (Krol et al. 2019).

Midwives have a key role in helping parents develop sensitivity and responsiveness to their developing baby, encouraging them to talk to and stroke their baby in response to movements, bolstering their confidence and highlighting the significance of their unique connections. Additionally, if the midwife perceives that there may be potential difficulties for the new parents to adjust to their role, she will inform the health visitor and refer the woman to a parenting programme for additional support, whilst continuing to act as a role model and source of positive parenting information.

It is particularly important that midwives do not perpetuate the old wives' tales that are counterproductive to engendering sensitive parenting. For example, 'don't pick him up, you'll make a rod for your own back', etc. We now know that close contact with parents who respond to their baby's cues enhances the baby's brain development and social behaviour long term (Gardner & Deatrick 2006). It is also important not to attribute purposeful intention to the baby who is crying or does not sleep through the night. Describing babies as 'naughty', 'good' or 'mischievous' perpetuates the myth that they are displaying a behaviour that needs fixing or is undesirable. Their requirements to feed frequently and be held close is a human need with evolutionary purpose, not the actions of a baby who wants to deliberately upset its parents.

ADVERSE CHILDHOOD EXPERIENCES

There are many additional parental factors that can impact on the quality of parental relationships with their baby. The families most at risk are those where there is domestic violence, substance abuse and enduring mental health problems. Those parents that have themselves experienced trauma as children may have developed personality disorders and go on to have disrupted attachments with their children and the cycle continues. Whilst it is recognised that interventions in childhood can help redress some of the damage caused by exposure to trauma and distress in childhood, prevention is better than cure and therefore to give every child the best start in life, intervention should begin before conception and continue throughout childhood (Early Intervention Foundation 2018:7). The Royal College of Psychiatrists (2018) recommend that preventing adverse childhood experiences (ACEs) must be core to national strategy and that expanding the provision of perinatal mental health services is needed to provide support for partners and fathers.

BECOMING A MOTHER

When thinking about the process of becoming a mother it is important to consider the social context in which such a transition is taking place. Traditionally, although not exclusively, women in mid-twentieth-century Britain had courted, married and left home (and often employment) before entering the sphere of mother-hood. However, today motherhood comes is myriad shapes and forms; it can happen after a long-standing relationship, secure employment and financial security; or as part of a happy, or not-so-happy, accident, which threw two people together who might never have previously contemplated having any future connection. Women sometimes become mothers again in a new relationship after a previous relationship breakdown and families can be a complex mix of children from both sides of the union as well as products of the new one.

Midwives need to make relationships with women quickly but securely. In antenatal clinics with 15-minute appointments, time is of the essence and she needs to establish who she is talking to in a consultation, without making assumptions or jumping to conclu-sions. For example, when a man and woman come into the con-sulting room together and there appears to be a large age gap, many midwives have fallen foul of presuming the accompanying man is the woman's father. Equally, the woman may be in her forties accompanied by a younger man; so, the midwife would be better informed and more able to provide personalised care if she made a friendly inquiry such as 'and you are?' before she causes any insult or irreparable damage to her relationship with the women.

The language of parenting is changing as the shape of families continue to evolve. LGBTQ parenting refers to lesbian, gay, bisexual, transgender and queer people raising children through a range of means including: donor insemination, IVF, surrogacy and adoption. The woman in the previous scenario may be a surrogate mother for a male couple, for example. Some lesbian wives take it in turn to have the children, so making a polite 'is this your first baby?' might get a mixed response. Increasingly there are reports of transgender people having babies and also enjoying the joys and challenges of parenthood (Trebay 2008). It is crucial that midwives do not marginalise people by failing to recognise the importance of the language they use; much better to ask, find out and understand than assume.

CHANGING IDENTITY

Erikson (1968) explored the concept of identity postulating that it is a way of describing oneself that comprises and amalgamates previous, current and future self-perceptions. However, according to Josselson (1987) there are significant gender differences and women often make meaning about their own identity through their accomplishments within relationships, especially with family. As individuals we all have hopes and aspirations but how these are manifest depends on our relationships with others in social groups and institutions. In an increasingly networked world our communications can transcend continents and identities become ethereal; it is human nature to connect with others and never more so than in the context of birth. Such connections are multiple and complex: between partners, woman to midwife, mother to infant.

Becoming a mother provides a new perspective on life. Priorities change but that does not mean that other roles become subordinate. For example, mothers often learn skills of organisation, negotiation and prioritisation that can enrich their other roles as employees, daughters and members of the community. New parenthood is a time when there can be a realisation of the magnitude of love their own parents have for them. Conversely, it may also raise emotions about connections with other family members, a time for reflection and flux. Appreciating the complexity that being a mother and protecting and investing in your child brings can add a greater sense of empathy with others juggling similar intricate and interwoven life challenges.

EXPECTED TO COPE

However, all is not rosy in the garden of parenthood. Most parents want to do the best for their babies and be seen to be doing so too. There is increasing pressure to be out and about with the new baby, with the latest pram and matching accessories. One woman in the PINK study (Baston 2006) talked about the expectation that as a new mother you are just expected to 'come home and carry on as normal [...] be a good wife, keeping the house tidy' and that 'it's such a fast roller coaster that nobody stops to sort of think, "well are you [ok]?"' She remembered that at her postnatal visits to the health visitor she answered the Edinburgh Postnatal Depression Scale (EPDS) questionnaire with the responses she felt she should give rather than how she actually felt. She went on to say:

> Everybody's there with their pristine babies, and you're taking them every week to get weighed, and they're asking 'how are you doing?' and you think, 'oh, I'm doing alright' but there's probably a lot of women who say they are and they're not really. I think there's so much expectations on you to be able to cope (Baston 2006:90).

Parents who are socially and economically disadvantaged may face challenges that make their transition to parenthood more difficult, including: higher levels of stress, less stable marital and parent–child relationships and less social support (Narciso et al. 2018). Whilst the former can cumulatively increase the risk of poorer emotional, social and cognitive development in the children, these effects can be cushioned by parents who have a developed capacity to understand their children's emotional states leading to empathy and secure attachment (Stacks et al. 2014). The midwife can assist parents in their transitions, help prepare them for the realities, joys and challenges of parenting.

SELF-ESTEEM

The next level of Maslow's model is the need for humans to be respected and feel valued. Self-esteem is defined as 'a favourable or unfavourable attitude towards the self' (Rosenberg 1965:15) and is considered to influence many other psychological concepts including personality, behaviour and clinical conditions such as anxiety and depression. Self-esteem is both a *trait*, an established and enduring personality characteristic, and a *state* that has a normal variation and may be short term.

SELF-ESTEEM AND MOTHERHOOD

A mother with high self-esteem herself is best placed to facilitate the development of high self-esteem in her infant by adopting a more sensitive and less controlling parenting style than women with low self-esteem (Bugental & Johnston 2000). As a sense of self-worth, parental contact and devoted attention during early childhood has an important impact on how a child feels loved and lovable. This investment of time and reciprocity given by parents forms a firm foundation for the child to develop and grow in confidence as it faces the inevitable challenges of becoming an adult.

Self-esteem changes throughout life's course, being high in children then decreasing towards adolescence when previously positive self-perceptions as an infant are replaced by evaluation of the self, based on feedback from others and comparison with peers. It then rises steadily throughout adulthood peaking at around the age of 60 years before beginning a sharp decline in older age (Robins & Trzesniewski 2005). It is an important concept to consider in relation to childbirth for a range of reasons. High self-esteem can be a predictor for positive relationships and general health and well-being (Orth & Robins 2014).

The development of new responsibilities such as partner, wife and mother are key events that influence and structure a person's position in their social context. The evaluation of these roles and their impact on self-esteem is mediated by perceptions of control and agency, and the emotional states of shame and pride, which influence the way that events are ultimately internalised (Robins & Trzesniewski 2005). Whilst there is some evidence that generally women experience a drop in self-esteem after childbirth and early motherhood (Bleidorn et al. 2016) becoming a mother is also an opportunity to experience meaning in life and develop a sense of mastery (Van Scheppingen et al. 2017). Ultimately, how a woman's self-esteem is influenced by the birth of her child will also be influenced by transitions in other life domains such as relationships, employment and age.

SUPPORTING MATERNAL AGENCY

The role of the midwife in supporting an environment where the woman feels she has control and a direct influence on the course of events is key. Feeling in control of what staff are doing, being treated with respect and being involved in decision-making are related to a positive childbirth experience and emotional well-being (Green & Baston 2003). Client-centred, personalised care is central to current UK maternity strategy (National Maternity Review 2016).

There are many opportunities throughout pregnancy, birth and motherhood where the midwife can boost a woman's self-confidence, whether its commenting on the amazing job she is doing growing and nurturing her baby; how powerful her body is during labour; or how her breastfeeding has contributed to baby's weight gain. A heightened state of self-worth and supporting a woman to find her own solutions can contribute to how a woman evaluates herself; self-esteem per se, however, cannot be given, it must be cultivated by the woman.

MOTHERHOOD AND THE MEDIA

Fluctuations in self-esteem can arise as the mother compares herself to those around her. Becoming a mother involves changes in the way a woman looks physically and how she looks at herself and is seen by others. Mothers are judged and judge themselves against the portrayals of 'good mothers' in the media, cultural expectations and peer social norms. Women give birth in a world where society holds many different constructs of what success in life looks like. The depiction in the media of women who are back in their size-10 jeans the week after birth, with perfect hair and make-up, paints an unrealistic picture of what it means to most parents, where nurturing and caring for a young baby takes all their attention and time, leaving little time for grabbing a shower, never mind donning Lycra and heading off down the gym.

BREASTFEEDING AND THE MEDIA

There are many emotive issues that are related to becoming a parent, what equipment to buy, what nappies to use and juggling childcare with going back to work. However, none of these match the emotions generated when the issue of breastfeeding is raised. The media debates include criticising midwives for promoting breastfeeding and for 'shaming' women into breastfeeding along with chastising women for feeding in public, etc. (see Resources). Globally women, parents and professionals continue to be bombarded by formula milk advertising, which is limited to varying degrees by the International Code of Marketing Breastmilk Substitutes.

MOTHERHOOD AND MENTAL HEALTH

ANTICIPATING BIRTH

The following vignette illustrates the impact of other women's experiences of labour and birth on a woman's own hopes, fears and expectations. These stories are even more potent when they are personal and relate to a family member or close friend. Mandy's story depicts a scenario whereby her mother's 'need' to have surgical births diminished her faith in her own body to rise to the challenge of physiological birth:

> My own mother had three caesarean births, the first an elective procedure, the second (me) an emergency caesarean followed by a further elective caesarean. As a child, I remember hearing stories about my birth, how dreadful an experience it had been and how my mother thought 'my baby must be dead'. She had suffered a protracted labour and received no information about her progress. She described her carers as cruel and her experience remains vivid over 50 years later. When I was pregnant with my first baby I was already a midwife. I hoped for a natural birth with no intervention. However, when I went into labour and 'failed to progress' despite regular contractions, I opted for an epidural in the 'knowledge' that a caesarean was on the cards. My mother's experiences lowered my threshold for belief in my body's ability to give birth unaided. In the event, I had an instrumental birth and subsequently had a spontaneous vaginal birth three years later.
>
> Mandy, midwife and mother, UK

There is often confusion in maternity circles regarding the impact of women's expectations for the birth. Some experienced midwives and obstetricians perpetuate the myth that women who have high expectations for the birth are 'setting themselves up to fail'. However, a groundbreaking multi-site study, *Great Expectations* (Green et al. 1998), clearly demonstrated that positive expectations are associated with positive experiences. This prospective study was particularly important because it asked women detailed questions about their expectations for the birth; for example, in relation to pain relief, interventions and involvement in decision-making etc., *antenatally*. It is human nature to temper one's aspirations in the light of what happened, therefore the questions about what women would like to happen at the birth should be answered antenatally, before the emotions of her experience can influence her evaluation of events.

The antenatal questionnaire discerned between what women wanted and what they actually expected to happen. Women were able to be realistic about the fact that, for example, they would have 'quite liked' to have been cared-for in labour by a midwife whom they had already met and to have that midwife with them at all times, but said that 'it probably won't happen'. Multivariate analyses concluded that:

> In every single case where there is a significant difference between women with high and low expectations it is the women with high expectations who have the better psychological outcome and women with low expectations who have the worst (Green et al. 1998:215).

FEAR OF BIRTH

Not all women can anticipate birth positively. Some women experience a severe fear of childbirth or tokophobia (Aksoy et al. 2015). According to a systematic review and meta-analysis (O'Connell et al. 2017), approximately 14 per cent of pregnant women worldwide have tokophobia, which is a phenomenon that is increasing. Symptoms include avoidance thoughts and behaviours to the extent that woman may put off becoming pregnant for many years or remain childless. It is more common in women expecting their first baby and those who have low self-esteem, anxiety and low partner and social support (Calderani et al. 2019). Tokophobia can be primary in women who do not have children, or secondary in response to a previous traumatic event. It is difficult to quantify how much tokophobia contributes to a request for caesarean birth for non-medical reasons, as some fear may relate specifically to fear of vaginal birth. A systematic review (Olieman et al. 2017) reports a rate of 1–9 per cent although the subsequent impact on maternal health is unclear.

MENTAL HEALTH MATTERS

Mothers support and sustain family life and without them children are at risk, therefore maternal mental health is an important factor in the fabric of society. We have already seen in relation to maternal mortality that the ultimate price of severe mental ill health on women and the impact of suicide of the families left behind is immeasurable. There is a range of postnatal illness that women can experience from mild to moderate anxiety and depression to acute psychosis. Some illnesses such as obsessive-compulsive disorders and post-traumatic stress disorder (PTSD) can become enduring and debilitating without the appropriate care and treatment.

Oakley (1980) offered a model for postnatal depression based on a woman's reaction to the significant life event of birth and the many associated changes that go with it: loss of income, change in identity, institutionalisation, change in physical appearance and occupational changes. She also considered the cumulative impact of interventions in labour, which ultimately led to separation and detachment from their infant. That events in labour could impact on women's emotional well-being became the subject of further research and is now widely acknowledged (Baston 2006).

The long-term impact of maternal depression on the cognitive development of the child, especially when it is prolonged, is well established (Goodman et al. 2011). The accessibility of another emotionally available adult, such as the father or other family members, can help protect the child from long-term sequelae. It is important that where feasible, mothers with severe mental illness are cared-for in facilities where they can maintain close contact with their babies.

However, whilst poor parental mental health can be a risk factor for a child's cognitive and emotional development, good parental mental health can help mitigate the impact of negative childhood experiences (Early Intervention Foundation 2018).

> Social and emotional skills are initially nurtured through a secure attachment relationship. Parents and caregivers foster attachment security through parenting behaviours that are predictable, sensitive and responsive to the child's needs. Feelings of attachment security allow children to develop positive expectations of themselves and others (Early Intervention Foundation 2018:11).

PRETERM BIRTH AND MENTAL HEALTH

Mothers who undergo preterm birth are more likely to experience postnatal depression and PTSD than women who have their baby at term (Anderson & Cacola 2017). Indeed, maternal mental ill health is a risk factor for preterm birth. Factors contributing to these outcomes include the initial shock and stress of having the baby earlier than expected as well as feelings of loss and grief (Yaari et al. 2019). Women who are socially disadvantaged are particularly at risk of psychological distress, following preterm birth, due to the impact on employment and the extra financial and emotional strain they face.

SELF-ACTUALISATION

From Maslow's point of view, self-actualisation is when an individual has achieved fulfilment at the highest level. They have become the best that they can be, are creative and are psychologically robust people. The linear path that Maslow described, however, does not always reflect real life, especially that of a mother. There will be times in anyone's life when we dip down from a place of success and achievement to rock bottom, perhaps following the death of a close partner or loss of employment.

The exhilaration of giving birth, holding the new baby that has been grown and protected by her body, might well be the pinnacle of all achievements. One woman from the PINK study (Baston 2006:132) recalls four years after the birth of her daughter:

> I mean I could have climbed a mountain, I could have flown off an Empire State Building, you could have done, you could have done anything. You know, you had suddenly, it was like, it's real. [...] I know you had all that time to think about it, but until you actually saw the whites of its eyes, you know, it was just, it wasn't real. But it was amazing.

The relief of her baby successfully negotiating the birth process as well as surviving it herself can be exhilarating. Sadly, not all women have this experience of becoming a mother. Consider teenage motherhood, for example; the scenario of a 15-year-old girl holding her new baby might represent a very different picture. Still a child herself, she may not have experienced the love and security she needs to feel safe. She may not have a place of sanctuary where she can focus on caring for her baby while others care for her.

Her pregnancy may have meant that she left school before achieving her academic potential. Conversely, however, the teenage mother may have planned her pregnancy and ultimately achieved a place of self-actualisation where she feels truly fulfilled, loved and accomplished. She may have broken free from the restrictions of 'childhood' and entered a new role where she is the most important player in the health and well-being of her child.

The reality of motherhood and the journey required to get there means that each individual woman's experience will be unique to her. Maternity services must continue to strive to provide care that is not only safe, but life-enhancing, personal and responsive. The impact of pregnancy, birth and postnatal care on a woman has long-lasting effects and creates memories that last a lifetime. The factors that impact on her appraisal of events are multi-factorial and culturally determined (Baston et al. 2008). That said, rigorous and regular evaluation of women's experiences may elucidate themes that can be used by services to continually improve their offer (Redshaw et al. 2019).

It has also been argued that midwives who work to the full extent of their role can also achieve self-actualisation (Court & Stevens 2009). Midwives who are able to provide antenatal, labour and postnatal care to a small caseload of women, for example, have the capacity to provide continuity of care, engage with families and develop enduring relationships. When working as truly autonomous practitioners with supportive colleagues, they share decision-making with women in partnership and experience a sense of agency and control; this is job satisfaction and role fulfilment at its peak.

CONCLUSION

The road to motherhood can be smooth, rocky or impossible to navigate depending on where you are born, live and work. Globally countless women face challenges that blight their path. Without access to the basic human needs of safe water, safe homes and access to skilled healthcare and life-saving interventions, many women will never reach the heady heights of self-actualisation. The role of the midwife has been demonstrated to be a life-changing intervention that has the potential to reduce maternal and infant mortality and make a significant impact on wider population health. At an individual level, the midwife also makes an important contribution to the lives of each and every woman she cares for. Being a kind and compassionate, knowledgeable companion throughout pregnancy and beyond, the midwife has the capacity to enhance the lives of future generations.

RESOURCES

Breast crawl, http://breastcrawl.org/science.shtml. Photos of the various stages of how the baby can self-attach at the breast supported by links to the research evidence to support this practice.

BREASTFEEDING IN THE MEDIA

Infant and young child feeding. World Health Organization, www.who.int/en/news-room/fact-sheets/detail/infant-and-young-child-feeding Important key facts about global breastfeeding rates, and recommendations to support increased rates across the world.

International Code of Marketing of Breastmilk Substitutes, www.unicef.org.uk/babyfriendly/baby-friendly-resources/international-code-marketing-breastmilk-substitutes-resources/guide-to-working-within-the-code/.

'Midwives told they must respect mothers who decide not to breastfeed' (*The Independent*, 12 June 2018), www.independent.co.uk/news/health/breastfeeding-midwife-royal-college-advice-mothers-bottle-feeding-respect-a8395041.html.

'Midwives should stop trying to shame new mothers into breastfeeding' (*Manchester Evening News*, 12 June 2018), www.manchestereveningnews.co.uk/news/greater-manchester-news/midwives-breastfeeding-bottle-feeding-shamed-14772775.

'New mothers should not be shamed into breastfeeding' (*Telegraph*, 12 June 2018), www.telegraph.co.uk/news/2018/06/11/new-mothers-should-not-shamed-breastfeeding/.

Magical Hour, www.magicalhour.org/aboutus.html Evidence-based information and photographs depicting the behaviour of newborn infants in the first hour after birth.

NCT first 1,000 days, new parent support, www.nct.org.uk/about-us. The NCT provide a range of opportunities for parents to understand more about pregnancy, childbirth and parenting.

Royal College of Midwives. Caring for you campaign, www.rcm.org.uk/supporting/getting-help/caring-for-you/. A resource for midwives to improve the resilience and well-being of the midwifery workforce.

Wider determinants of health (2017), www.youtube.com/embed/eF7ZstmCgVs. Video explaining the impact of the social determinants of health.

REFERENCES

ACOG (American College of Obstetricians and Gynecologists) (2018). How your fetus grows during pregnancy. www.acog.org/Patients/FAQs/How-Your-Fetus-Grows-During-Pregnancy?IsMobileSet=false. Accessed 8 November 2019.

Aksoy A, Ozkan H, and Gundogdu G (2015). Fear of childbirth in women with normal pregnancy evolution. *Clin Exp Obstet Gynecol* 42:179–183.

Anderson C, and Cacola P (2017). Implications of preterm birth for maternal mental health and infant development. *MCN: The American Journal of Maternal/Child Nursing* 42(2):108–114.

Ballard O, and Morrow A (2013). Human milk composition: nutrients and bioactive factors. *Pediatr Clin North Am* 60(1):49–74.

Baston H (2006). Women's experience of emergency caesarean birth. PhD thesis. University of York, http://etheses.whiterose.ac.uk/14082/.

Baston H, Rijnders M, Green J, et al. (2008). Looking back on birth three years later: factors associated with a negative appraisal in England and in the Netherlands. *Journal of Reproductive and Infant Psychology* 26(4):323–339.

Betran A, Torloni M, Zhang J, et al. (2015). What is the optimal rate of caesarean section at population level? A systematic review of ecologic studies. *Reprod Health* 12:57.

Bleidorn W, Hopwood C, Lucas R, et al. (2016). Life events and personality trait change. *Journal of Personality* 86(1), doi:10.1111/jopy.12286. Accessed 24 November 2019.

Boatin A, Schlotheuber A, and Betran A (2018). Within country inequalities in caesarean section rates: observational study of 72 low and middle income countries. *BMJ* 360, www.bmj.com/content/bmj/360/bmj.k55.full.pdf.

Boerma T, Ronsmans C, Dessalegn Y, et al. (2018). Global epidemiology of use of and disparities in caesarean sections. *Lancet* 392(10155):1341–1348.

Brimdyr K, Cadwell K, Stevens J, et al. (2017). An implementation algorithm to improve skin-to-skin practice in the first hour after birth. *Maternal & Child Nutrition* 14(2), doi:10.1111/mcn.12571.

Bugental D, and Johnston C (2000). Parental and child cognitions in the context of the family. *Annu Rev Psychol* 51:315–344.

Byrom S, and Downe S (2015). Introduction: what's going on in maternity care? In *The roar behind the silence: why kindness, compassion and respect matter in maternity care* (ed. Byrom S and Downe S). London: Pinter and Martin Ltd.

Calderani E, Giardinelli L, Scannerini S, *et al.* (2019).Tocophobia in the DSM-5 era: outcomes of a new cut-off analysis of the Wijma Delivery Expectancy/Experience Questionnaire based on clinical presentation. *J Psychosom Res.* 116:37–43.

CDC (Centers for Disease Control and Prevention) (2006, updated 2012). Principles of epidemiology in public health practice. 3rd ed. U.S. Department of Health and Human Services, www.cdc.gov/csels/dsepd/ss1978/SS1978.pdf.

Coad J (2011). *Anatomy and physiology for midwives*. 3rd ed. Edinburgh: Churchill Livingstone.

Court C, and Stevens T (2009). Relationship and reciprocity in caseload midwifery. In *Emotions in midwifery and reproduction* (ed. Hunter B and Deery R). Basingstoke: Palgrave Macmillan.

Crenshaw, JT (2014). Healthy birth practice #6: keep mother and baby together – it's best for mother, baby, and breastfeeding. *J Perinat Educ.* 23 (4):211–217.

Cusick S, and Georgieff M (2019). The first 1,000 days of life: the brain's window of opportunity. UNICEF, www.unicef-irc.org/article/958-the-first-1000-days-of-life-the-brains-window-of-opportunity.html. Accessed 21 November 2019.

Devis P, and Knuttinen M (2017). Deep venous thrombosis in pregnancy: incidence, pathogenesis and endovascular management. *Cardiovasc Diagn Ther.* 7(Suppl 3): S309–319.

Early Intervention Foundation (2018). Realising the potential of early intervention, www.eif.org.uk/files/pdf/realising-the-potential-of-early-intervention.pdf. Accessed 21 November 2019.

Elejalde R, and Giolito E (2019). More hospital choices, more C-sections: evidence from Chile. Discussion paper. IZA Institute of Labor Economics, http://ftp.iza.org/dp12297.pdf.

Erikson E (1968). *Identity: youth and crisis*. New York: Norton.

EWEC (Every Woman Every Child) (2015). The global strategy for women's, children's and adolescents' health (2016–2030), www.everywomaneverychild.org.

Gardner M, and Deatrick J (2006). Understanding interventions and outcomes in mothers of infants. *Issues in Comprehensive Pediatric Nursing* 29(1):25–44.

Green J, Coupland V, and Kitzinger J (1998). *Great expectations: a prospective study of women's expectations and experiences of childbirth*. Hale: Books for Midwives Press.

Green J, and Baston H (2003). Feeling in control during labor: concepts, correlates, and consequences. *Birth* 30(4):235–247.

Goodman S, Rouse M, Connell A, *et al.* (2011). Maternal depression and child psychopathology: a meta-analytic review. *Clinical Child and Family Psychology Review* 14:1–27, doi:10.1007/s10567-010-0080-1.

Holt-Lunstad J, Robles T, and Sbarra D (2017). Advancing social connection as a public health priority in the United States. *Am Psychol.* 72(6):517–530, doi:10.1037/amp0000103.

Homer C, Friberg I, Dias M, *et al.* (2014). The projected effect of scaling up midwifery. *The Lancet* 384(9948):1146–1157.

Hoope-Bender P, de Bernis L, Campbell J, *et al.* (2014). Improvement of maternal and newborn health through midwifery. *The Lancet* 384 (9949):1226–1235.

ICM (International Confederation of Midwives) (2011, updated 2017). International definition of the midwife, www.internationalmidwives.org/assets/files/definitions-files/2018/06/eng-definition_of_the_midwife-2017.pdf. Accessed 9 November 2019.

Josselson R (1987). *Finding herself: pathways to identity development in women.* San Francisco, CA: Jossey-Bass.

Kee W (2005). Confidential enquiries into maternal deaths: 50 years of closing the loop. *BJA: British Journal of Anaesthesia* 94(4):413–416, doi:10.1093/bja/aei069.

Kitzinger S (1983). *The new good birth guide.* London: Penguin.

Knight M, Bunch K, Tuffnell D, *et al.* (eds) on behalf of MBRRACE-UK (2018). Saving lives, improving mothers' care – lessons learned to inform maternity care from the UK and Ireland confidential enquiries into maternal deaths and morbidity 2014–2016. Oxford: National Perinatal Epidemiology Unit, University of Oxford, www.npeu.ox.ac.uk/downloads/files/mbrrace-uk/reports/MBRRACE-UK%20Maternal%20Report%202018%20-%20Web%20Version.pdf.

Krol K, Moulder R, Lillard T, *et al.* (2019). Epigenetic dynamics in infancy and the impact of maternal engagement. *Science Advances* 5(10), doi:10.1126/sciadv.aay0680.

Marmot M (2010). Fair society, healthy lives: the Marmot review. Institute of Health Equity, www.instituteofhealthequity.org/resources-reports/fair-society-healthy-lives-the-marmot-review/fair-society-healthy-lives-full-report-pdf.pdf.

Marmot M (2017). Marmot indicators briefing. Institute of Health Equity, www.instituteofhealthequity.org/resources-reports/marmot-indicators-2017-institute-of-health-equity-briefing/marmot-indicators-briefing-2017-updated.pdf.

Maslow A (1943). A theory of human motivation. *Psychological Review* 50 (4):370–396, http://psycnet.apa.org/record/1943-03751-001.

Modig K, Berglund A, and Talbäck M (2017). Estimating incidence and prevalence from population registers: example from myocardial infarction. *Scandinavian Journal of Public Health* 45(17):5–13.

Narciso I, Relvas A, Ferreira L, *et al.* (2018). Mapping the 'good mother' – meanings and experiences in economically and socially disadvantaged contexts. *Children and Youth Services Review* 93:418–427.

National Maternity Review (2016). Better births: improving outcomes of maternity services in England, www.england.nhs.uk/wp-content/uploads/2016/02/national-maternity-review-report.pdf.

NHS Digital (2019). NHS maternity statistics, https://digital.nhs.uk/data-and-information/publications/statistical/nhs-maternity-statistics/2018-19.

NICE (National Institute for Health and Care Excellence) (2008a, updated 2014). Maternal and child nutrition PH11, www.nice.org.uk/guidance/ph11.

NICE (National Institute for Health and Care Excellence) (2008b, updated 2019). Antenatal care: for uncomplicated pregnancies, CG62, www.nice.org.uk/guidance/cg62/chapter/1-Guidance. Accessed 18 April 2019.

Oakley A (1980). *Women confined: towards a sociology of childbirth.* Oxford: Martin Robertson.

O'Connell MA, Leahy-Warren P, Khashan AS, *et al.* (2017). Worldwide prevalence of tocophobia in pregnant women: systematic review and meta-analysis. *Acta Obstetricia Et Gynecologica Scandinavica* 96(8):907–920.

Olieman R, Siemonsma F, Bartens M, *et al.* (2017). The effect of an elective cesarean section on maternal request on peripartum anxiety and depression in women with childbirth fear: a systematic review. *BMC Pregnancy Childbirth* 17 (1):195.

Orth U, and Robins R (2014). The development of self-esteem. *Current Directions in Psychological Science* 23(5):381–387.

O'Sullivan A, Farver M, and Smilowitz J (2015). The influence of early infant-feeding practices on the intestinal microbiome and body composition in infants. *Nutr Metab Insights* 8(Suppl 1):1–9, doi:10.4137/NMI.S29530.

Part K, Moreau C, Donati S, *et al.* (2013). Teenage pregnancies in the European Union in the context of legislation and youth sexual and reproductive health services. *Acta Obstetricia Et Gynecologica Scandinavica* 92(12):1395–1406.

PHE (Public Health England) (2018). A framework for supporting teenage mothers and young fathers, https://assets.publishing.service.gov.uk/government/uploads/system/uploads/attachment_data/file/796582/PHE_Young_Parents_Support_Framework_April2019.pdf. Accessed 10 November 2019.

PHE (Public Health England) (2019a). Physical activity for pregnant women, https://assets.publishing.service.gov.uk/government/uploads/system/uploads/attachment_data/file/829894/5-physical-activity-for-pregnant-women.pdf.

PHE (Public Health England) (2019b). Child and maternal health data, https://fingertips.phe.org.uk/profile/child-health-profiles/data#page/1/gid/1938133225.

PMNCH/WHO (2018). Partnership for maternal, newborn & child health report: commitments to the every woman every child global strategy for women's children's and adolescents' health (2016–2030), www.everywoma neverychild.org/wp-content/uploads/2018/09/commitments-report-2015-2017.pdf.

Redshaw M, Martin C, Savage-Mcglynn E, *et al.* (2019). Women's experiences of maternity care in England: preliminary development of a standard measure. *BMC Pregnancy and Childbirth* 19(1):1–13, doi:10.1186/s12884-019-2284-9.

Renfrew MJ, McFadden A, Bastos HM, *et al.* (2014). Midwifery and quality care: findings from a new evidence-informed framework for maternal and newborn care. *The Lancet* 384(9948):1129–1145, doi:10.1016/S0140-6736 (14)60789-3.

Robins R, and Trzesniewski K (2005). Self-esteem development across the life span. *Current Directions in Psychological Science* 14(3):158–162.

Robson MS (2001). Classification of caesarean sections. *Fetal and Maternal Medicine Review* 12(1):23–39.

Robson SJ, and de Costa C (2017). Thirty years of the World Health Organization's target caesarean section rate: time to move on. *Med J Aust* 206 (4):181–185.

Rosenberg M (1965). *Society and the adolescent self-image.* Princeton, NJ: Princeton University Press.

Royal College of Psychiatrists (2018). Written evidence from Royal College of Psychiatrists, http://data.parliament.uk/writtenevidence/committeeevidence. svc/evidencedocument/health-and-social-care-committee/first-1000-days-of-life/written/88926.html.

Stacks A, Muzik M, Wong K, *et al.* (2014). Maternal reflective functioning among mothers with childhood maltreatment histories: links to sensitive parenting and infant attachment security. *Attachment & Hum Dev* 16 (5):515–533.

Tamburini S, Nan S, Han W, *et al.* (2016). The microbiome in early life: implications for health outcomes. *Nature Medicine* 22(7):713–722.

Tommy's (2019). Premature birth statistics, www.tommys.org/our-organisa tion/why-we-exist/premature-birth-statistics. Accessed 8 November 2019.

Trebay G (2008). He's pregnant. You're speechless. *New York Times,* 22 June,www.nytimes.com/2008/06/22/fashion/22pregnant.html. Accessed 22 November 2019.

UNICEF/WHO (2018). Database of skilled health personnel, based on population-based national household survey data and routine health systems data, https://data.unicef.org/wp-content/uploads/2018/02/Interagency-SAB-Dat abase_UNICEF_WHO_Apr-2018.xlsx.

United Nations (2019). Sustainable development goals. Goal 3: ensure healthy lives and promote well-being for all ages, www.un.org/sustainabledeve lopment/health/.

Uvnäs-Moberg K, Ekström-Bergström A, Berg M, *et al.* (2019) Maternal plasma levels of oxytocin during physiological childbirth – a systematic review with implications for uterine contractions and central actions of oxytocin. *BMC Pregnancy Childbirth* 19(285), doi:10.1186/s12884-019-2365-9.

Van Lerberghe W, Matthews Z, Achadi E, *et al.* (2014). Country experience with strengthening of health systems and deployment of midwives in countries with high maternal mortality. *The Lancet* 384(9949):1215–1225, doi:10.1016/S0140-6736(14)60919-3.

Van Scheppingen M, Denissen J, Chung J, *et al.* (2017). Self-esteem and relationship satisfaction during the transition to motherhood. *Journal of Personality and Social Psychology* 114(6):973–991, doi:10.1037/pspp0000156.

Wise J (2018). Alarming global rise in caesarean births, figures show. *BMJ* 363, doi:10.1136/bmj.k4319.

WHO (World Health Organization) (2015). WHO statement on caesarean section rates, https://apps.who.int/iris/bitstream/handle/10665/161442/WHO_RHR_15.02_eng.pdf?sequence=1.

WHO (World Health Organization) (2017a). WHO recommendations on antenatal care for a positive pregnancy experience, https://apps.who.int/iris/bitstream/handle/10665/250796/9789241549912-eng.pdf?sequence=1.

WHO (World Health Organization) (2017b). Programme reporting standards for sexual, reproductive, maternal, new-born, child and adolescent health. Geneva: (WHO/MCA/17.11), https://apps.who.int/iris/bitstream/handle/10665/258932/WHO-MCA-17.11-eng.pdf;jsessionid=6F07BA27D486DCFA149C5B35AD718A84?sequence=1.

WHO (World Health Organization) (2019). Trends in maternal mortality 2000 to 2017: estimates by WHO, UNICEF, UNFPA, World Bank Group and the United Nations Population Division. Geneva, www.who.int/reproductivehealth/publications/maternal-mortality-2000-2017/en/.

WHO CSDH (Commission on Social Determinants of Health) (2008). Closing the gap in a generation, www.who.int/social_determinants/final_report/csdh_finalreport_2008.pdf.

Yaari M, Treyvaud K, Lee K, *et al.* (2019). Preterm birth and maternal mental health: longitudinal trajectories and predictors. *Journal of Pediatric Psychology* 44(6):736–747.

THE ROLES OF THE MIDWIFE

There are many ways to describe the multiple facets of the midwife's role. This book uses a patchwork model approach to depict the role in seven distinct elements that are closely and seamlessly aligned. This is to demonstrate the many aspects of the midwife's daily transitions; however, in reality they merge and overlap in a much more complex way. This chapter begins with the international definition of a midwife to summarise what a midwife does. It then introduces the patchwork model and provides a summary of how the seven elements capture the main facets of the midwife's role. It then goes on to use the Nursing and Midwifery Council's Code (NMC 2018) as a framework to illustrate how these key components interface and overlap. Examples of women's narratives from the PINK study (Baston 2006) will be used to illustrate their perceptions of care during childbirth.

DEFINITION

The International Confederation of Midwives (ICM 2017) provides an overarching definition of the midwife that includes that she has completed an approved education programme and met the required level of competence to be registered or licenced to practise in that country. The 'Scope of Practice', or what the midwife can actually do, is succinctly summarised as follows:

> The midwife is recognised as a responsible and accountable professional who works in partnership with women to give the necessary support, care and advice during pregnancy, labour and the postpartum period, to

conduct births on the midwife's own responsibility and to provide care for the newborn and the infant. This care includes preventative measures, the promotion of normal birth, the detection of complications in mother and child, the accessing of medical care or other appropriate assistance and the carrying out of emergency measures.

The midwife has an important task in health counselling and education, not only for the woman, but also within the family and the community. This work should involve antenatal education and preparation for parenthood and may extend to women's health, sexual or reproductive health and child care. A midwife may practise in any setting including the home, community, hospitals, clinics or health units (ICM 2017:1).

The first part of this statement includes the key to all of midwifery practice; that the midwife is 'with women' and works in partnership with them always. The woman needs to be listened to and heard, with the midwife making no judgement about the woman's values or beliefs. We are all different, and have unique priorities and therefore cannot assume that the values we hold as important will be held in the same esteem by others. This ICM definition captures the extended reach of the midwife, from before conception to maternal and infant public health; not only 'with women' but also 'with community'.

THE ROLES OF THE MIDWIFE – INTRODUCTION TO THE PATCHWORK MODEL

PROFESSIONAL – ACCOUNTABLE AND SAFE

Professionalism is central to the role of the midwife, as illustrated by the patchwork model (see Figure 2.1); it underpins all other roles. According to the NMC, professionalism is 'characterised by the autonomous evidence-based decision making by members of an occupation who share the same values and education' (NMC 2016:3). It is about inspiring confidence in others, both patients and colleagues, to work to a high standard of competence and integrity.

First and foremost, the midwife needs to work in such a way that she does no harm and provides safe care. Since its inception, the

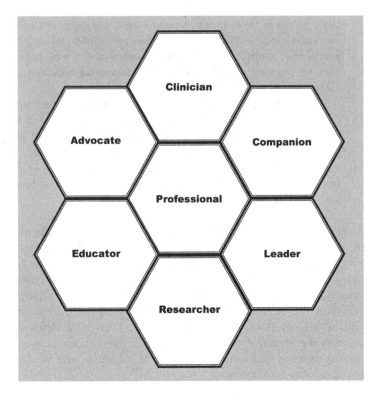

Figure 2.1 The midwife's role: patchwork model

professional role of the midwife has been clearly defined and laid down in various documents produced by the professional body. Over time this has been simplified and the essence of all registrants (nurses, midwives and nursing associates) is encapsulated in one comprehensive bible of standards which underpin all professional practice. The Code (NMC 2018) details the standards that are expected of the midwife, in whatever setting and role she performs – 'they are not negotiable or discretionary' (NMC 2018:3).

The title of the midwife is protected in UK law and it is an offence for someone to work in this capacity, proclaiming they hold such a qualification, when they are not entitled to do so (NMC 2017). The midwife has a central role in facilitating and coordinating care between members of the multi-professional team, working collegiately with them. She continually updates her knowledge and shares that with others to uphold the reputation of the midwifery profession. For a brief history of the birth and development of the midwifery profession, see Chapter 3.

CLINICIAN – SKILLED AND COMPETENT

One of the many great things about becoming a midwife is the opportunity to combine clinical dexterity with critical appraisal skills. It is as though the eyes, hands and brain are linked in such a way that the midwife has special detection skills, able to 'know' when something is not quite right. Of course, this is a romantic notion – in actual fact, the midwife is observing, hearing, smelling, feeling and combining the many fragments of data to create a picture that makes sense. When a piece of information is slightly obscured, the picture created is distorted and alarm bells sound. The midwife may not be able to 'put a finger on it' but will know that further exploration is needed.

To make clinical judgements and wise decisions the midwife needs to able to use all of these senses. In situations of stress or distraction, hunger or fatigue, the midwife's judgement can be compromised and she may miss vital pieces of evidence to support intuitive care. Thus, the midwife needs to undertake self-care to ensure her competence is maintained.

Perceptions of competence and believing that staff know what they are doing is fundamental to women trusting their judgements. It is part of our socialisation to trust the 'professionals' and some women come into the maternity care system with a very clear perception that staff are the experts. The following quotes from women in the PINK study (Baston 2006) illustrate how women assess the competence of the staff who care for them:

> They were all competent at what they were doing. And I think you put a lot of trust in them because you don't know what you're doing. You know you've never had a baby before, and they've seen babies come and go, it's their job, and so they're used to babies. And so you just sort of you trust them (166).

When staff demonstrate that they know what they are doing this helps alleviate the potential fear that could be caused because of the circumstances and being cared for by staff they do not know:

> I don't think anybody introduced themselves to me ... but that didn't bother me, 'cos they just seemed to work really well as a team, they all had their little job to do [...] they just seemed really organised and I just felt really happy that I was in good hands really, erm, at that point, I didn't feel worried by that at all (167).

Staff can also demonstrate competence when they act quickly in response to an obstetric emergency. It is important to women that the staff do not hesitate when swift action is necessary:

> I couldn't have wanted people to react more quickly and positively, and they obviously knew their job, and they knew what was happening [...] I think had there been a little bit more procrastination about 'what am I going to do?' I'd have started to think. 'oh, what are you going to do/what's happening?' But they were just, it was 'no, this is what we're going to do, and this is why' and erm, ok (166).

Women are very quick to pick up on signs of incompetence. Hesitation, lack of eye contact and avoiding the question are responses that create chinks in the midwife's professional armour.

COMPANION – COMMUNICATING AND NURTURING

To be truly 'with women' midwives need to demonstrate compassion. There are various levels of engaging with women. We first need to have either asked an appropriate question or listened to a woman's spontaneous narrative to hear what she is saying. On one level we might feel pity, for example, if a woman has had a previous difficult experience, which we can elevate to expressions of sympathy when we articulate our concern. Empathy involves seeing the situation from their perspective and sharing their emotions whilst compassion involves action and the desire to make things better and alleviate their suffering (Burton 2015).

It takes time to learn some skills, and generally women understand that a midwife is junior and needs to practise. Women appreciate that sometimes procedures are difficult or painful. However, it is the manner in which procedures are performed that makes all the difference. Failure to acknowledge that further expertise is required or that they are causing discomfort is not forgivable. One woman in the PINK study described her experience of catheterisation:

> And it was so painful, and erm she didn't apologise for it being painful it went on for a long time, and then she just went and got someone else who did it immediately, she was using the wrong size catheter or something. And I was upset about that, that you know, someone would carry on trying even though it was painful, and I'm not someone who would scream out and say ... she didn't seem to look at me and sort of see that it was very painful (168).

Being approachable and friendly is particularly valued by women. One woman in the PINK study, when asked if there was anything she might like to say to staff who care for women in labour, said:

> When they (sighs) when the people are actually in sort of labour and are obviously getting to the stage when they are going for epidural and things, just make sure that they are as reassuring as possible, and as normal as possible. Try and forget they're medics and just (laughs slightly) be themselves, you know what I mean, 'cos sometimes when a midwife's being a midwife, (pause: 2 seconds) she's being too much like a, a nurse if you like. And not enough like someone who's there who need, you know, will help you (175).

ADVOCATE – PROTECTING AND ENABLING

The Code (NMC 2018:7) states that the midwife, as a registrant, should 'Act as an advocate for the vulnerable, challenging poor practice and discriminatory attitudes and behaviour relating to their care'. Whilst there are legal advocacy roles in the realm of social care and looking after people with disabilities, the same principles apply to the midwifery setting, whereby women should have access to someone who will listen to their point of view and speak or act on their behalf when necessary.

Women can be or become vulnerable at any point of their pregnancy journey. For example, a woman who has experienced previous sexual abuse and has disclosed this to her midwife may have been reassured that she will not be exposed to intimate examinations by a male obstetrician. The midwife, as her advocate, must ensure that this arrangement is followed through, even if it means referring to a senior colleague to facilitate it in practice. During labour, when a woman may be in pain and fearful, the midwife will continue to ensure that care reflects the woman's aspirations, wherever possible.

On rare occasions the midwife may observe care that is not best practice. For example, if she sees that a baby is about to be separated from its mother, so that she can be transferred to the ward, the midwife can intervene and demonstrate how this can be achieved safely, without interruption to skin-to-skin contact. By acting as a role model, she can protect the health and well-being of mothers and babies in her care.

The midwife will demonstrate advocacy at the individual level and also at a wider organisational and population level, being the voice of the childbearing women in the way that services are configured and women are represented. This may involve engagement with local community groups and the Maternity Voice Partnership (MVP) to garner feedback from women about any proposed changes or review of maternity care delivery.

EDUCATOR – FACILITATING LEARNING

So much of what the midwife does is about empowering women to be involved in decisions about their care. To be able to do this, midwives engage in a range of informal and formal educational opportunities with women and their families. Much of this work is in relation to ensuring that women know how to monitor their own health and well-being during pregnancy. For example, the midwife can use the opportunity when checking a woman's blood pressure, to ask her if she is experiencing any headaches or visual disturbances. She can inform her what to do if she does and why it is important.

A useful model to consider when thinking about what elements a woman might need to consider when being asked to undertake a particular action or change of behaviour, such as stopping smoking, is that suggested by Michie et al. (2011). The COM-B model, where B stands for 'Behaviour', relates to:

- **C**apability – does she have the skills and knowledge to stop smoking? 'can't'
- **O**pportunity – has she been referred to the smoking cessation team? 'don't'
- **M**otivation – does she understand the implications of continuing to smoke? 'won't'

To raise a woman's motivation, by informing her that an issue is really important, but without giving her the opportunity or ensuring she has the capability, can be counterproductive. Women need to have all three elements in order to make a sustainable behaviour change.

Midwives are also key players in promoting a learning culture for their colleagues wherever they work. It can be formally through mandatory updates and conference feedback or opportunistically such as sharing snippets of information from Twitter or research papers across the multidisciplinary team. Midwives also learn from their students and being a mentor in the clinical environment provides a great opportunity to hear about the latest research evidence from their junior colleagues. All registrants are required to undergo a formal process of 'revalidation' (NMC 2019) to demonstrate their continuous learning and this is described in more detail later in this chapter.

Being a reflective practitioner and learning from events where things went well or could have been better is an essential part of developing professional wisdom. For this continuous scholarship to be effective midwives need to be able to both give constructive feedback and receive it from others.

RESEARCHER – CREATOR OF NEW KNOWLEDGE

Midwives in clinical practice will come across many opportunities to ask questions about the best way to deliver a particular element of care, how women experience it and what are the attitudes of staff providing it. Developing research skills begins early in the pre-registration journey as student midwives learn how to appraise research papers and assess the quality of published papers. They then learn how to assimilate that evidence and incorporate it into a narrative to support or refute a particular aspect of practice. Gaining in confidence, student midwives can begin to include evidence in the options they are giving women. For example, the Birthplace Study (Hollowell et al. 2011) concluded that for healthy women with uncomplicated pregnancies, giving birth in midwifery-led units was safe for babies and led to fewer interventions for mothers. Women have a right to this knowledge and need it in order to make informed decisions about their care.

Having the opportunity to undertake primary research as a midwife is a privilege. However, it takes determination and drive to overcome the many hurdles involved. These challenges include: formulating a coherent idea, applying for funding, having setbacks and enabling others to understand the value that research brings to the care of women. It can also be conflicting for the midwife to be objective when she is collecting data, as the following vignette demonstrates.

REFLECTIONS OF A MIDWIFE RESEARCHER

I found that undertaking the interviews evoked both positive and negative emotions. Of particular note was the diversity of social circumstances. Many interviewees lived in cramped accommodation, whereas others enjoyed luxurious surroundings. Only one woman did not live with a partner, and some worked around childcare. I reflected on how isolated and unsupported some women appeared compared with others who were able to pursue a busy social schedule. Each baby was growing up within unique 'family units' exposed to a range of social opportunities and threats. Some of these children played noisily and creatively during the interview, others gazed relentlessly at a television screen. Although I wore my 'researcher' hat and asked my questions objectively, listening attentively to the responses, I wonder if and how my emotions were conveyed in my body language. As an experienced midwife, I would like to think that I am able to walk into anyone's house, intuitively appreciate a woman's particular situation and care for her appropriately. However, as a researcher, I was not in a position to use the information I gleaned in the same way (Baston 2006:185).

There is a potential danger that midwives can fail to notice outmoded practices that might be staring them in the face, because they are so familiar with providing care in a certain way. The idea of looking through a different lens or wearing different hats can be useful when aiming to take an objective stance and see things from an alternative perspective.

LEADER – CHANGE AGENT

In relation to this aspect of the midwife's role, leadership is about being able to influence change, being respected and being able to inspire others. These are qualities that can be seen at all levels of midwifery, from student midwife to the most senior level in the organisation. Above all, the midwife who aims to ensure that clinical practice and the care that women receive is the best it can be needs to be able to communicate effectively. She needs to able to articulate her ideas and insights in a way that is meaningful to those she hopes to influence.

Midwives who demonstrate leadership also need to be good team players. They need to be able to empathise with their colleagues and understand the pressure they face when undertaking particular aspects of their role. At a very simple level, for example, if a midwife identifies that a particular process is outdated or ineffective, when considering alternatives, she would need to consider who it might affect, what the cost implications might be and whom she needs to engage to illicit a meaningful change.

For maternity services to meet the needs of the women and families they serve, they need to continually evolve in the light of new technologies, changing consumer expectations and societal values. Midwives therefore need to embrace change and be optimistic about the future, rather than clinging on to what they learned when they were students. A clinical 'comfort zone' should only be one where practice is safe and effective and delivered with sensitivity and compassion, not a place where care is based on tradition and inertia.

THE CODE AND THE MIDWIFE

The Code (NMC 2018) presents the fundamental standards which all midwives must uphold in their professional practice. One of its key principles is that whoever the registrant is, they must work within the limits of their competence, which means in practice that they should not do anything that they have not had the training to perform or are not personally and professionally competent to undertake. This also includes any skill that they have acquired since registration, over and above those basic standards expected of someone of the same area of practice.

The Code is in four domains:

1   Prioritise people
2   Practice effectively
3   Preserve safety
4   Promote professionalism and trust

Each domain comprises a range of statements and these will be referred to throughout this chapter in relation to the role of the midwife.

DOMAIN 1 – PRIORITISE PEOPLE

TREAT PEOPLE AS INDIVIDUALS AND UPHOLD THEIR DIGNITY (1)

As with all caring situations, when the midwife meets a woman for the first time and in subsequent appointments and events, what she knows about her background, life experiences, hopes and fears is limited. In order to get by in life we often use stereotypes to help us understand a particular situation, but in so doing, we make assumptions that may not apply to the individual in front of us. Green et al. (1990) have argued that using stereotypes, for example, that an uneducated, working-class woman has no aspirations that birth will provide emotional fulfilment, can be misleading and inappropriate and can be a poor substitute for effective communication. It is therefore essential that the midwife makes every possible effort to get to know the individual woman and what her particular needs might be. Women must be given every opportunity to express their individuality and have their unique values upheld wherever possible.

When considering the issue of dignity, it might seem obvious that midwives have a key role in ensuring that women's modesty and privacy are maintained throughout all encounters with her. Pregnancy and childbirth are extremely exposing processes and there are many times when intimate examinations, which professionals perform day in and day out, can lead a woman to feel extremely vulnerable. Again, the midwife may have no idea what previous experiences she may have had, such as childhood sexual abuse or domestic violence, and cannot assume that this will be a straightforward event for her.

Upholding a woman's dignity is further reaching than the physical side of care; it includes ensuring that care is given with kindness and compassion. It means that she should not be kept waiting and that she receives a response to meet her needs without unnecessary delay. All members of the care team should respect the woman's personal space and ask permission to undertake any aspect of care, no matter how seemingly trivial it might feel to them.

LISTEN TO PEOPLE AND RESPOND TO THEIR PREFERENCES AND CONCERNS (2)

Listening is an active process which can be an acquired skill. When student midwives are first starting out on their journey to becoming a fully fledged midwife it can be quite difficult not to be overwhelmed by the task in hand and what to do next, rather than actually hearing what a woman is saying. Learning to pick up on cues that women give during interactions with them is essential for a trusting relationship; reading between the lines of what a woman is actually saying and then checking this interpretation with her.

Midwives must acquire insight into how their responses can impact on a woman's experience. This was eloquently highlighted in groundbreaking work by Mavis Kirkham (1989) where she identified that during conversations with women, some midwives block a woman's request for information by talking in platitudes; a phenomenon she described as 'verbal asepsis' (125). In the PINK study, this was brought home when a woman interviewed four years after the index birth experience said how frustrated she was because no one took her fears about her second birth seriously:

> Everybody, every antenatal I, I, I mean, in fairness I, we moved, so I changed midwives. But they both still sort of said the same, 'oh, don't worry, no two births are the same. You'll be absolutely fine.' [...] And

> then everybody said, 'oh no, you know, you'll be fine, and it'll be a
> much better experience' and, and then you know, you, it's not is it?
> 'Cos it's, it all went wrong again (87–8).

The midwives who heard the worry and fear expressed by this woman could have responded by finding out more about what had happened previously and what might help her feel better about the impending birth.

Part of the listening and getting to know women is understanding how much involvement they want in decisions about their care. There is no black and white with this issue; a woman may wish to defer all emergency decisions to her carers, but still be totally involved in other aspects such as intrapartum pain relief or positions in labour. Again, not making assumptions is essential and offering the woman information and encouraging her to think about what would be most appropriate for her particular situation is the ideal route to take.

On occasions, a woman refuses an aspect of care that might prevent a poor outcome. For example, a woman may decline any offers of smoking cessation support or decline to come into labour ward for assessment following an episode of reduced fetal movements. On such occasions, the midwife must take every reasonable step to ensure the woman has information that she understands, in order to make such decisions. For example, with the issue of smoking, if she had not been informed about the increased risk of miscarriage, premature birth or stillbirth associated with smoking in pregnancy, then her decision to decline the offer of support is not truly 'informed'. So, part of the midwife's role is to offer information, make sure the woman has grasped the key messages and document the care she has given. The door should always be open for the woman to change her mind.

MAKE SURE THAT PEOPLE'S PHYSICAL, SOCIAL AND PSYCHOLOGICAL NEEDS ARE ASSESSED AND RESPONDED TO (3)

One element of the midwife's role is helping women achieve a healthy pregnancy and to use the opportunity to have a stock check on their current lifestyle and health status. Pregnancy is often described as a 'teachable moment' (Phelan 2010) where women are open to having conversations they would otherwise avoid, such as about their weight. This window of opportunity is short during a pregnancy and so the midwife needs to be careful that she works in partnership with the woman, finds out what she already knows about a particular health issue and then offers her tailored information that she can access easily. Giving blanket information to all women is inappropriate, while, making sure that there is equity, there does need to be an element of signposting everyone to where they can get further information and making detailed plans for those who have an immediate health need.

ASSESSMENT

A holistic approach to a woman's circumstances means that the midwife is aware of the factors that might prevent her accessing a particular aspect of care. For example, if a woman is living in poverty and she is unable to afford the bus fare to the big supermarket where food is cheaper, her food choices will be limited and her diet will therefore be reflective of what she can afford locally. To be able to take such factors into account the midwife conducts a comprehensive booking interview (see Chapter 5) when she first meets the woman in early pregnancy. This includes her medical, obstetric (previous pregnancies and birth outcomes) and social history as well as her current health and emotional well-being. However, there is limited value in collecting all of this information if it then does not inform subsequent plans. Together, the woman and midwife can discuss what, when and how additional support can be identified and accessed.

ACT IN THE BEST INTEREST OF PEOPLE AT ALL TIMES (4)

When women are accessing maternity care, it is a fundamental principle that they should be consulted, involved and in agreement with all plans for care. So, for example, a woman should know what blood tests have been taken, when to expect the result and what might happen if the result is not within normal parameters. This sounds simple, yet when women access health services, it is very easy for them to adopt a 'patient role' and acquiesce to all options offered to them. The midwife needs to make sure that the woman's best interests are always served, and make every effort to ensure that the woman understands the implications of her choices. Even signed consent, if gained from a woman who does not have the full information, is not 'informed' and is not legal.

There are circumstances in healthcare where it is not possible to seek or gain informed consent from a woman. This may be if she is unconscious when admitted to a maternity unit, following a major haemorrhage, for example. In such an event, it would be appropriate for the obstetric team to take her for emergency surgery and even perform a hysterectomy, without her consent, as it would be in her 'best interest' to save her life. There are also situations when a woman might be fully conscious but unable to make decisions about her care, because she 'lacks capacity'. This may be due to a learning disability or a mental health crisis and there are comprehensive laws and legal process that protect women in such circumstances. The midwife therefore needs to keep informed regarding how these are translated into local guidance and ensure that the correct procedures are adhered to.

The Code also seeks to protect the interests of staff involved in care delivery. It clearly states that in situations where a member of staff has a conscientious objection to a particular procedure, for example, medical termination of pregnancy, that they inform their manager, colleagues and the individual receiving care and arrange for another appropriate person to care for her.

RESPECT PEOPLE'S RIGHT TO PRIVACY AND CONFIDENTIALITY

Healthcare provision take place in a complex web of information about individuals; this is personal data that women have a right to expect it be kept safe and only the appropriate people have access to it. Information may be held in a range of platforms, including electronic databases, paper or digital records. Women should be aware of the routine sharing of data, such as between the midwife and health visitor and what would require additional permission in line with the current legal framework.

Being a midwife means having access to a wide range of information about people; where they live, their medical history and their current treatment. Inevitably there are times when a midwife comes across a woman she may already know, such as an old school friend or a neighbour. All midwives must be vigilant in ensuring that they never discuss a woman's care with anyone else outside the healthcare setting; pregnancy and birth are particularly sensitive issues and it can be detrimental to a woman's social circumstances if third parties were inadvertently made aware of details of event. Similarly, the midwife must not access the woman's data in order to find out information about acquaintances or even family members; this would be a breach of confidentiality and a disciplinary offense.

There are times, however, when a midwife should and must share information in order to protect her safety or that of the public. If a woman discloses that she is having suicidal thoughts, for example, the midwife should inform her that she will share that information with a mental health practitioner who can further assess the woman's health status. Other circumstances where the midwife might have information about a potential safeguarding or child protection issue, for example, would necessitate prompt sharing with the appropriate agencies. The midwife should always be able to account for her decision where information was shared and clearly document her actions.

DOMAIN 2 – PRACTISE EFFECTIVELY

ALWAYS PRACTICE IN LINE WITH BEST EVIDENCE (6)

Whilst desirable, this standard is not always achievable. This is not because midwives do not want to give evidence-based practice (EBP), but because there may be limited evidence about what is best practice in a particular circumstance. The availability and use of evidence will vary depending on the discipline, but a recent estimate of EBP in primary care (Ebell et al. 2017) concluded that only 18 per cent of doctors' decisions were based on evidence.

Maternity care led the way with evidence-based practice and the collation of systematic reviews in the groundbreaking compendium *A Guide to Effective Care in Pregnancy and Childbirth*, by Enkin et al. (1989). Ian Chalmers and colleagues founded the Cochrane Collaboration in 1993 (Higgins & Green 2008), with the aim of conducting and disseminating reviews of randomised controlled trials (RCTs). Cochrane systematic reviews are seen as the gold standard 'go-to' source of information, which are conducted following a strict protocol and highlight where further research is needed. A simplified explanation of their function is that they pull together the body of evidence on a particular aspect of practice, grade the studies for quality, then pool the results of RCTs on the same subject. Ultimately recommendations for practice are made, carefully framed by the limitations the reviewers identified. Not all areas of clinical midwifery lend themselves to being investigated by an RCT, however. Would it be ethical, for example, to randomise women to have either an elective caesarean or await natural events, and thus expose women to potentially unnecessary surgery?

In a caring profession like midwifery, there are also many questions around what impacts on a woman's experience of a particular element of care, what makes her feel safe, valued and involved. This may require in-depth investigation of her feelings and perceptions, with contextual background information painting a rich picture of her lived experience. This qualitative, theory-building research requires very different methods and study design, involves fewer numbers and more words. Ideally, an issue is examined using a mixed method approach to capture and identify how best to provide treatment and care, to provide new knowledge that is meaningful to midwives. It is just as important to know if a treatment is acceptable to women as it is to know if it works.

Implementing new evidence in practice can be challenging. Practitioners become comfortable with providing care in the way that they were first taught. NHS trusts invariably have their own 'guideline group' or means of articulating national and professional guidance within a local framework. Local guidelines provide a 'this is how we do it here' but should reflect contemporary evidence and therefore have a structured programme for review. This work is often overseen by a governance lead who can keep a watchful eye on the review cycle, or indeed expedite review if there has been a marked change in national guidance. All new guidance should come with a package of education and audit to ensure that it becomes truly embedded in care pathways.

The Code makes it clear that midwives are responsible for not only maintaining their clinical skills, but also adapting as new technologies and products come into play. Employers are also responsible for ensuring that learning opportunities are made available to staff to support safe and effective care.

To care for women and their families, midwives must be able to communicate effectively and in a way that best meets their needs. When people access health services they are often under the influence of adrenaline, making it difficult to concentrate and take in information. Midwives must therefore avoid using jargon, or overly complicating a message, whilst ensuring that enough information is provided to support understanding and rational decision-making. This may mean taking a step back occasionally and confirming what the woman understands by a particular test, for example. The midwife may need to use additional visual aids or written information to support what she is saying. The use of touch in communication must take account of what is culturally appropriate.

When women do not speak English or have a limited understanding there should be support mechanisms in place to provide adequate translation. This may be telephone or web based, but ideally a professional, face-to-face interpreter using the same language and dialect. It is considered poor practice to use family members or children as interpreters as it is impossible to know what message has been conveyed when sensitive, confidential information is being discussed.

WORK CO-OPERATIVELY (8)

Healthcare workers need to collaborate and co-operate for the common good of providing skilled and appropriate care. This means that they need to communicate effectively and regularly with each other and recognise the contribution that each other has in the provision of holistic woman-centred care. Midwives are the experts in maternity care when a woman and her baby are well. They can identify when their condition changes and should not hesitate to refer to a more senior colleague when appropriate.

There are many means by which colleagues can keep each other appraised of a woman's particular circumstances; directly by talking, remotely by digital interfaces such as electronic whiteboards or through the written word. It is essential that detailed plans for care are made so that each professional concerned is aware of their role and when to seek additional advice.

There need to be mechanisms whereby if a midwife is not satisfied with a particular course of action her colleague is suggesting or recommending, that this can be escalated to a more senior person. Whilst the midwife should be supportive of the colleagues she works with, this should not be at the expense of public safety.

SHARE YOUR SKILLS, KNOWLEDGE AND EXPERIENCE FOR THE BENEFIT OF PEOPLE RECEIVING CARE AND YOU COLLEAGUES (9)

We all need feedback about the way we behave and perform to enable us to learn and develop. This means we should provide it to others by praising good practice and reflecting when things do not go so well. As registrants, midwives are required to collect feedback from a range of sources, such as families, preceptors, mentors, managers and peers. Feedback should always be given in a constructive way, with offers of support to develop and enhance women's care.

Feedback must always be objective and supported by evidence to be of value. There need to be examples to substantiate any concern; it should not be third-hand or influenced by subjective hearsay. Given the opportunity, most people can grow in knowledge, skills and confidence, but if battered by relentless, unhelpful negative feedback, can become demotivated and defensive.

KEEP CLEAR AND ACCURATE RECORDS RELEVANT TO YOUR PRACTICE (10)

As outlined in Standard 7, communication between professionals is paramount. The Code recognises the midwife's legal accountability to keep accurate records of care and stipulates that they should be made as soon after an event as possible (contemporaneous) to ensure accuracy. If, because of an emergency situation or during a birth, it is physically impossible to be 'with woman' and 'with record' at the same time, the midwife should make note of the timing of key events and record them as soon after the event as possible. Midwifery records are a legal document and should be accurate, legible and unaltered.

Increasingly midwives are documenting their care in a digital format. To do so requires they use a unique 'login', which provides an audit trail of the care that has been given. It is important that midwives do not make entries under another colleague's login, as they would then be unable to provide evidence that it was they who had given care. Keeping data safe is a modern-day challenge; it can be inadvertently stolen, corrupted or shared risking a breakdown in communication or breach of confidentiality.

BE ACCOUNTABLE FOR YOUR DECISIONS TO DELEGATE TASKS AND DUTIES TO OTHER PEOPLE (11)

Midwives work as part of a multi-professional team and therefore share the care of women with many other professionals and support staff. If a task is delegated this should only be to a person with the correct level of knowledge and skills to perform it effectively. This may mean that the person to whom the task has been delegated has some supervision and that feedback and support is given as needed. The standard of care should remain high and no member of staff should ask another member of staff to undertake a task they had not been trained to do, or indeed, accept a task that is outside the scope of their competence.

HAVE IN PLACE AN INDEMNITY ARRANGEMENT THAT PROVIDES APPROPRIATE COVER FOR ANY PRACTICE YOU TAKE ON AS A NURSE, MIDWIFE OR NURSING ASSOCIATE IN THE UNITED KINGDOM (12)

When a midwife works for an NHS trust the employer provides insurance via vicarious liability. However, to comply with this arrangement means that the midwife must fulfil the requirements of her employment, which as a registrant means upholding the standards of the Code. Midwives are entitled to work independently of the NHS but must have appropriate insurance cover. Such indemnity should cover them in the event of being involved in the care of a woman or baby where there is a poor outcome. Because of the potential for harm to occur during the childbirth continuum and for that harm to have lifelong implications for a child in terms of being dependent on carers or loss of potential earnings, independent insurance cover must be substantial as a claim for damages may result in a payout in excess of millions of pounds. Similarly, the legal fees required to defend such a claim would be significant and being a member of a professional organisation is prudent.

DOMAIN 3 – PRESERVE SAFETY

RECOGNISE AND WORK WITHIN THE LIMITS OF YOUR COMPETENCE (13)

Midwives are the experts in caring for pregnant, birthing and postnatal women, in circumstances where the mother and her baby are well. When everything is straightforward the midwife will remain the lead professional throughout a woman's journey. However, if there is a deviation from the norm, if the mother or the baby show signs of compromise, the midwife must access the clinical expertise of an appropriate practitioner. This was eloquently articulated in 'Maternity Matters' (Department of Health 2007) when it was stated 'All women will need a midwife and some need doctors too' (15), and this principle is maintained in current doctrine. It is of the utmost importance for women's safety that professionals work together and ensure they refer appropriately as soon as a concern is identified. Even when a woman has been referred to another professional, the midwife will continue to coordinate her care and ensure that the required treatment is carried out.

To be able to recognise when the physical or mental health of the woman is worsening, the midwife must be able to undertake a range of clinical assessments and use her professional judgement to identify a problem. She will need to know the parameters of normality and, when her findings fall outside of these, how to act without delay. There are circumstances, such as in an emergency, when the midwife's actions can make the difference between life and death or life and serious compromise. Learning how to summon help, initiate resuscitation and coordinate the team are skills that develop with experience but also need regular refreshment in line with new evidence. Midwives must make themselves available to access mandatory training to ensure that they maintain and develop their competence.

BE OPEN AND CANDID WITH ALL SERVICE USERS ABOUT ALL ASPECTS OF CARE AND TREATMENT, INCLUDING WHEN ANY MISTAKES OR HARM HAVE TAKEN PLACE (14)

Midwives have a professional 'duty of candour', which means that they must make women and families aware if there have been untoward incidents that have put the mother or baby at risk. Explanations should be open and honest, timely and made in such a way that the women understand the consequences. When such incidents are serious in nature, such disclosure should be escalated to the senior midwifery and obstetric team, as a junior midwife may not be aware of all of the contributing factors and the impact in the individual case.

ALWAYS OFFER HELP IF ANY EMERGENCY ARISES IN YOUR PRACTICE SETTING OR ANYWHERE ELSE (15)

Whilst it is a professional expectation that a midwife will always assist at situations she comes across, such as a woman unexpectedly birthing outside of hospital, she must only act within the limits of her competence. She should summon help and assistance as she would in a maternity care setting, continue to provide basic life support where necessary and exercise emotional intelligence at all times. Any care or assistance that is given by midwives should not compromise their own safety or jeopardise that of others.

ACT WITHOUT DELAY IF YOU BELIEVE THAT THERE IS A RISK TO PATIENT SAFETY OR PUBLIC PROTECTION (16)

Midwives often find themselves working in situations that feel demanding and sometimes stressful. Where a midwife works in a maternity unit, there will usually be access to other colleagues and peers to provide a second opinion or offer a helping hand. However, sometimes, because of the unpredictable nature of birth and maternity events, there will be occasions when the workload becomes too heavy, either in terms of the number of women and babies that need to be cared for, or because of the complexity of the situation. In such circumstances, the midwife must escalate her concerns about a situation to a senior colleague so that extra help can be found.

When basic standards of safety are compromised the midwife has a duty to raise her concerns. Equally, the midwife must not interfere or prevent a colleague from doing so and, if in a senior role, should protect those affected from harassment, after a concern has been raised. NHS Trusts recognise the importance of enabling staff to speak up if they have a concern. Historically known as 'whistle blowing', when an employee speaks out against their own organisation, it is now acknowledged that by supporting staff to voice their apprehensions, a culture of bullying and intimidation can be prevented, and proactive interventions can be made to avert potential disaster and patient harm. There is now a recognised role and network hosted by the Care Quality Commission (CQC 2019) of 'freedom to speak up guardians' whom staff can confide in if they have a public interest concern.

RAISE CONCERNS IMMEDIATELY IF YOU BELIEVE A PERSON IS VULNERABLE OR AT RISK AND NEEDS EXTRA SUPPORT AND PROTECTION (17)

Midwives have privileged positions; they see families in a range of social circumstances and sometimes see things they wish they had not. But the midwife has a duty to escalate any concerns she has where she suspects that someone might be at risk of harm through neglect or abuse. In such circumstances the midwife can and must share information with the relevant agencies in line with local guidelines. For example, if the midwife witnesses emotional or physical abuse by another to a woman in her care, she can escalate to the local social work duty team or designated safeguarding official.

ADVISE ON, PRESCRIBE, SUPPLY, DISPENSE OR ADMINISTER MEDICINES WITHIN THE LIMITS OF YOUR TRAINING AND COMPETENCE, THE LAW, OUR GUIDANCE AND OTHER RELEVANT POLICIES, GUIDANCE AND REGULATIONS (18)

Managing drug administration is a fundamental core aspect to the role of the midwife. Increasingly complex care and new pharmacologies mean that there are a range of drug regimens and protocols that need to be actioned, depending on a woman's individual circumstances. This is a complex arena, which the midwife begins to learn from day one of her undergraduate programme and ultimately will have responsibility for at the end of her midwifery education.

The midwife does not blindly follow instructions, and when coordinating the care of women and babies, needs to consider the whole picture. To protect client safety, midwives need to keep abreast of the latest recommendations regarding therapeutic doses and the circumstances in which certain medications are indicated. For example, it is recommended that women with a previous history of pre-eclampsia should take low dose aspirin daily from 12 weeks of pregnancy (NICE 2019). The midwife caring for a woman who fits this criterion must therefore ensure that the woman receives this information and is referred for an appropriate prescription. The midwife will continue to check compliance and ongoing monitoring of any issues related to this aspect of care throughout the woman's pregnancy.

Not only is the midwife responsible for identifying women who might benefit from a particular medication during their pregnancy, she is also required to act intelligently when administering medication prescribed by others. Human error is a challenge at any point within healthcare systems, and a midwife's role in protecting the public from harm means that any question about the appropriateness of a medication is explored. For example, is this safe for a woman who is allergic to penicillin, in the first trimester of pregnancy or if a woman is breastfeeding? Such questions such be addressed, even if the prescriber is a senior medical colleague; ultimately, midwives are responsible for their own actions.

MIDWIVES' EXEMPTIONS

There are a range of legal requirements around the prescribing and administration of drugs. Midwives cannot prescribe drugs unless they have undertaken an additional post-registration programme of education. However, they do have a bespoke range of drugs, which are known under the category of 'midwives' exemptions', that they are able to supply to a mother without a prescription by a doctor. These are common drugs that might be needed during the birthing process, such as oxytocin, which causes the uterus to contract and expel the placenta, or lidocaine, used as pain relief prior to perineal repair. They are called 'exemptions' because they are drugs for which there is an exemption clause in the Medicines Act 1968 (Government 1968:57) enabling midwives to supply medicinal products, as determined by the 'Health Minister'. The regulations that govern the application of the Act are outlined in schedule 17; the list of drugs, which is reviewed in light of contemporary practice, can be amended by the Secretary of State for Health and Social Care.

There is a quirk in the legislation in relation to how it applies to student midwives. According to part 3 of schedule 17 of the Human Medicines Regulations (Government 2012), a student midwife can administer the drugs in the exemption list, under the direct supervision of a midwife, except controlled drugs. So, where a midwife can administer morphine to a mother in labour without a prescription by a doctor, a student midwife cannot, although she can take part in the checking and preparation of it. A student midwife can, however, give the same drug, under the direct supervision of a midwife, if it had been prescribed by a doctor (NMC 2017:20–1). See the NMC document 'Practising as a Midwife in the UK' (NMC 2017:25–7) for the list of drugs to which the exemptions apply.

BE AWARE OF, AND REDUCE AS FAR AS POSSIBLE, ANY POTENTIAL FOR HARM ASSOCIATED WITH YOUR PRACTICE (19)

We have already considered some of the ways the midwife can protect the public from harm in relation to: using the best available evidence (Standard 6); fostering clear communication between colleagues (Standard 7); working co-operatively (Standard 8); accurate record keeping (Standard 10); appropriate delegation (Standard 11); working within the limits of professional competence (Standard 13); raising concerns about safety in the workplace (Standard 16); and safe drug administration and storage (Standard 18). This standard is advocating that the midwife also considers a whole system approach to reducing risk and learning from mistakes. For example, if a midwife made a drug error, whilst there would be a process around ensuring that appropriate action is taken, it would also be important to consider what might have contributed to that mistake. The Health and Safety Executive (HSE) describes these as Performance Influencing Factors (PIFs) (HSE 2019) and they relate to the job, person and organisations.

Elements of learning that might come from an error could include: ensuring that guidelines are up to date; midwives wear a tabard saying 'do not disturb – drug round in progress'; midwives are required to take breaks; mandatory learning opportunities are provided; and so on. In an organisation that encourages a no-blame culture and wants to learn from any errors made, it becomes everybody's business to adapt and respond as new and safer ways of practising come to light.

Maternity services have a track record with regard to highlighting the importance of preventing the spread of infection (see Chapter 3). Hospital-acquired infections are a source of morbidity and mortality, contributing to extended hospital stays, consumption of health service resources and personal misery. Every effort should be made to ensure that the woman does not develop a life-threatening infection as a result of the care she receives and that she is not put at risk of contracting an infection from another patient, relative or member of staff.

Midwives can take responsibility for reducing the risk of infection on a range of levels. From a personal perspective, for example, meticulous hand washing is essential before and after clinical contact with women, acting as a role model to parents by demonstrating such practice. Midwives can also act as role models to staff, women and visitors accessing the maternity unit, by using hand gels when entering the ward and disposing of contaminated waste in the appropriate bins. Women should also be encouraged to take personal responsibility for reducing their own risk of infection, washing their hands before and after changing their sanitary pads and after changing the baby's nappy.

From a public health perspective, midwives can ensure that they take up opportunities for seasonal flu vaccination and encourage others with small children, elderly relatives and people in risk groups to do the same. From a clinical perspective, midwives are involved in implementing guidelines that have been developed to reduce infection as a result of clinical and surgical interventions. Midwives should also make sure they use the equipment available to them to prevent their own exposure to infection, such as gloves, aprons and visors where appropriate.

DOMAIN 4 – PROMOTE PROFESSIONALISM AND TRUST

UPHOLD THE REPUTATION OF YOUR PROFESSION AT ALL TIMES (20)

It is expected that midwives will behave with honesty, integrity and lawfully, as befits someone in a caring profession. There is a certain level of dignity that is also expected from a midwife. Women trust midwives with their most personal information at times when they might feel vulnerable and out of control, such as during labour and birth. If midwives are seen behaving unprofessionally, then women may have concerns that their own circumstances might not be respected or treated confidentially. Whilst it is acceptable and indeed preferable that midwives have a relaxed relationship with the women in their care, this should remain on a professional basis at all times to enable objectivity to be maintained. Midwives should not let personal, religious or political beliefs cloud clinical professional judgement.

Midwives must continue to behave professionally when not at work. Maintaining confidentiality in all spoken, written and social media exchanges is essential; women and colleagues have a right to privacy and expect it to be upheld both during and after any professional contact. It should always be assumed, when having conversations outside of work, that someone connected to the person in question is within earshot or might somehow see a social media post that discloses their identity. Hence, it is simply best practice not to discuss work in public and never disclose a person's identity, even in private, one-to-one conversations.

Student midwives learn by observing and emulating midwives whom they feel project the appropriate attributes of their chosen profession. It is essential therefore that all midwives behave as mentors to the midwives of the future, as well as other associate professionals and support staff. For example, students who see a midwife treating domestic staff with respect and courtesy are more likely to value the essential contribution that all staff make to the care of women. For a midwife to care for a woman safely and in a timely way, there needs to be a clean room, appropriate equipment in working order, stocks of clean linen and the provision of fresh food and beverages; no midwife works in isolation – the assistance and input from all staff is invaluable.

UPHOLD YOUR POSITION AS A REGISTERED NURSE, MIDWIFE OR NURSING ASSOCIATE (21)

Women who have experienced fantastic care from their midwife and grateful relatives often want to show their appreciation and gratitude. However, midwives need to be careful not to accept gifts that might be construed as having an influence on the relationship. So, whilst it is fine to accept a box of chocolates or flowers, anything more substantial must be gracefully declined or returned. Relationship with clients must remain on a professional basis.

As midwives are generally held in high esteem, it might be assumed that they exercise good judgement when it comes to being able to recommend products or services outside the health service. However, giving recommendations is dangerous territory, which midwives need to avoid getting involved with, as what might appear to be a valuable product or useful service may in fact be less than optimum. For example, a midwife might recommend to a woman that she attends preparation for childbirth classes; however, other than an NHS-provided class, she should avoid advocating a particular person or company, because the midwife cannot vouch for their credentials, insurance status or outcomes. Women can be given general principles and then directed to explore the available options for themselves.

On occasions, particularly if there has been a new document released or event coming up, the media will want to have the views of a professional to provide insight and a sound bite. A typical situation might be if the media get to hear about activities relating to the International Day of the Midwife (5 May). However, the media want to create newsworthy copy and some journalists will take an interviewee away from the original topic in order to ask a more sensational question. It takes experience and nerve to deal with the press and a junior member of staff should defer all requests to a senior colleague, who will then consult with the Trust communications department before any such interaction takes place. Occasionally the Trust will invite the media, if it is in their best interest, such as if a new facility is being opened, but the terms and details of the communication will be closely supervised. Women or service users should only be involved if they consent to do so.

FULFIL ALL REGISTRATION REQUIREMENTS (22)

The Nursing and Midwifery Council set standards regarding how midwives achieve and maintain their status on the professional register. The standards for pre-registration midwifery education (NMC 2009, updated 2020) must be achieved by student midwives on completion of their programme of education and they must be maintained throughout the midwife's career. Each registration period of three years, midwives must undergo a process of revalidation (see www.revalidation.nmc.org.uk for details), which requires them to provide the NMC with assurance that they have:

- undertaken a minimum of 450 practice hours as a midwife;
- undertaken and provided evidence for 35 hours of continuous professional development (CPD), of which at least 20 must have included participatory learning;
- obtained five pieces of practice-related feedback from either women or colleagues;
- written five pieces of reflection relating to CPD, feedback or event in practice;
- a reflective discussion with another registrant;
- self-declared good health and character;
- professional indemnity; and
- confirmation of the above from line manager.

In addition to the above, midwives must keep their knowledge and skills up to date and learn new skills that might be required to undertake their role. For example, as technologies are constantly evolving, new online applications are becoming part of mainstream practice. No matter how senior or experienced a midwife is, it is essential for the provision of safe and effective care that new technologies are embraced. Digital documentation and e-prescribing, for example, are integral elements of care in many Trusts, and competence with these platforms is vital for care delivery.

Many elements of learning are mandatory for midwives to complete every year; these include emergency skills and drills, fire safety and many governance issues such as documentation and how to escalate concerns.

It is a professional expectation that midwives have a level of health that enables them to do their job in a safe and appropriate way. Whilst employers can make reasonable adjustments, when ill health arises, it is also expected that midwives contribute to their own health and well-being, making every effort to maintain physical and emotional health. Many NHS Trusts have a range of schemes available to employees, such as occupational health departments, mindfulness applications and workplace well-being schemes, to support staff to stay well.

CO-OPERATE WITH ALL INVESTIGATIONS AND AUDITS (23)

This standard requires registrants to assist the NMC with any audits or investigations that they need to conduct, including taking part in any hearings or providing witness statements, to enable their regulatory function to be fulfilled. Such reviews might be in relation to an individual's practice, such as examining training records, or disclosing a criminal offence. Also, when joining new employment, the midwife should disclose any previous restriction to their practice or disciplinary process.

Sadly, there are occasions when all does not go well with pregnancy and birth and midwives are asked to account for their actions or comment on the events that they were involved in. Most trusts have a clinical governance department and a lead for maternity-related issues who co-ordinate responses to complaints and investigate clinical incidents. Midwives should engage the support of their professional body, if an allegation is made against them, to gain support through the process of writing statements and engaging with the legal department. Being involved in an investigation is an extremely upsetting time for the midwife involved and the colleagues who are asked to provide evidence.

RESPOND TO ANY COMPLAINTS MADE AGAINST YOU PROFESSIONALLY (24)

It is unusual for midwives to receive complaints and it can therefore be an unsettling time. However, the midwife can also see this as an opportunity for development, to work with the feedback and enhance their knowledge and skills. The midwife should never let any complaint affect the care that she gives and the opportunity for another midwife to take over her care should be considered to avoid any potential for unease or embarrassment on either part.

PROVIDE LEADERSHIP TO MAKE SURE PEOPLE'S WELL-BEING IS PROTECTED AND TO IMPROVE THEIR EXPERIENCE OF THE HEALTH AND CARE SYSTEM (25)

Anyone can show leadership qualities, no matter how junior or inexperienced. A student midwife who questions why particular practice is performed, or challenges bullying behaviour, is a leader and agent of change. Qualified midwives must demonstrate effective leadership at all times; showing respect and empathy for the staff that they work with. Taking responsibility for careful management of resources, setting priorities and minimising risk are part of each midwife's daily repertoire. They must put women and their family's needs above their own, to ensure that quality care is provided.

CONCLUSION

The patchwork model illustrates the key component of the midwife's role. Professionalism is central to her work and the NMC Code provides guidance on how this can be achieved in clinical practice. The requirements of the Code are extensive and detailed providing a framework for the provision of safe, effective and personalised care. The midwife must uphold these standards and show leadership by supporting her colleagues to do the same.

RESOURCES

AIMS Association of Improvements in maternity Services, www. aims.org.uk. Provides an insight into the role of campaigning to protect the human rights of childbearing women.

Association of Radical Midwives (ARM), www.midwifery.org.uk/. A library and archive of resources for midwifery activists protecting professional independence in the UK.

Cochrane Library, www.cochranelibrary.com/ A searchable resource comprising a library of systematic reviews of randomised controlled trials.

Health and Safety Executive (2019). Risk – controlling the risks in the workplace, www.hse.gov.uk/risk/controlling-risks.htm.

Independent Midwives UK, https://imuk.org.uk/. Source or information about the role and practice of the independent midwife.

Royal College of Midwives (RCM), www.rcm.org.uk. The website for the professional body for midwives in the UK. It hosts a range of guidance and standards and learning resources for its members.

REFERENCES

Baston H (2006). Women's experience of emergency caesarean birth. PhD thesis. University of York, http://etheses.whiterose.ac.uk/14082/.

Burton N (2015). Empathy vs. sympathy. *Psychology Today*, 22 May, www.psychologytoday.com/gb/blog/hide-and-seek/201505/empathy-vs-sympathy. Accessed 26 October 2019.

CQC (Care Quality Commission) (2019). National Guardian's Office. www.cqc.org.uk/national-guardians-office/content/national-guardians-office.

Department of Health (2007). Maternity matters: choice, access and continuity of care in a safe service. London: Department of Health, https://webarchive.nationalarchives.gov.uk/20130103004823/http://www.dh.gov.uk/en/Publicationsandstatistics/Publications/PublicationsPolicyAndGuidance/DH_073312. Accessed 24 August 2019.

Ebell M, Sokol R, Lee A, *et al.* (2017). How good is the evidence to support primary care practice? *Evidence Based Medicine* 22(3):88–92.

Enkin M, Keirse M, Neilson J, *et al.* (1989). *A guide to effective care in pregnancy and childbirth*. New York: Oxford University Press.

Government (1968). Medicines Act 1968, www.legislation.gov.uk/ukpga/1968/67/pdfs/ukpga_19680067_en.pdf.

Government (2012, amended 2016). The Human Medicines (Amendment) Regulations 2016, https://www.legislation.gov.uk/uksi/2016/186/contents/made.

Green J, Kitzinger J, and Coupland V (1990). Stereotypes of childbearing women: a look at some evidence. *Midwifery* 6(3):125–132.

Higgins J, and Green S (eds) (2008). *Cochrane handbook for systematic reviews of interventions*. Chichester: John Wiley & Sons, www.academia.edu/39839676/Cochrane_Handbook_for_Systematic_Reviews_of_Interventions_THE_COCHRANE_COLLABORATION. Accessed 31 October 2019.

Hollowell J, Puddicombe D, Rowe R, *et al.* (2011). The birthplace national prospective cohort study: perinatal and maternal outcomes by planned place of birth. Birthplace in England Research Programme. Final Report Part 3. London: NIHR Service Delivery and Organisation Programme.

HSE (Health and Safety Executive) (2019). Performance influencing factors, www.hse.gov.uk/humanfactors/topics/pifs.pdf. Accessed 26 August 2019.

ICM (International Confederation of Midwives) (2017). International definition of the midwife, www.internationalmidwives.org/assets/files/definitions-files/2018/06/eng-definition_of_the_midwife-2017.pdf.

Kirkham M (1989). Midwives and information-giving during labour. In *Midwives, research and childbirth* (ed. Robinson S and Thomson AM). Boston, MA: Springer.

Michie S, Van Stralen M, and West R (2011). The behaviour change wheel: a new method for characterising and designing behaviour change interventions. *Implementation Science* 6(1):42, https://implementationscience.biomedcentral.com/track/pdf/10.1186/1748-5908-6-42.

NICE (National Institute for Health and Care Excellence) (2019). Hypertension in pregnancy: diagnosis and management. NG 133, www.nice.org.uk/guidance/ng133. Accessed 25 August 2019.

NMC (Nursing and Midwifery Council) (2009, updated 2020). Standards for pre-registration midwifery education, www.nmc.org.uk/globalassets/sitedo cuments/standards/nmc-standards-for-preregistration-midwifery-education. pdf. Accessed 26 August 2019.

NMC (Nursing and Midwifery Council) (2016). Enabling professionalism in nursing and midwifery practice, www.nmc.org.uk/globalassets/sitedocuments/ other-publications/enabling-professionalism.pdf. Accessed 2 November 2019.

NMC (Nursing and Midwifery Council) (2017, updated 2019). Practising as a midwife in the UK: an overview of midwifery regulation, www.nmc.org.uk/ globalassets/sitedocuments/nmc-publications/practising-as-a-midwife-in-the-uk.pdf. Accessed 25 August 2019.

NMC (Nursing and Midwifery Council) (2018). The Code: professional standards of practice and behaviour for nurses, midwives and nursing associates, www.nmc.org.uk/globalassets/sitedocuments/nmc-publications/ nmc-code.pdf. Accessed 16 August 2019.

NMC (Nursing and Midwifery Council) (2019). Revalidation: what you need to do, http://revalidation.nmc.org.uk/what-you-need-to-do.1.html. Accessed 26 August 2019.

Phelan S (2010). Pregnancy: a 'teachable moment' for weight control and obesity prevention. *American Journal of Obstetrics & Gynaecology* 202(2), doi:10.1016/j.ajog.2009.06.008.

MIDWIFERY – AN EVOLUTIONARY TALE

INTRODUCTION

Looking back in history and trying to make meaning from it is an inexact science. We all see the world through the lens of our experience and beliefs, which means that what we read is subject to variation in its interpretation. The magical nature of pregnancy and birth means that it has been enveloped in folklore and mythology, superstition and mystique. Examining the history of midwifery is therefore fraught with complexity. We need to understand the historical context of bygone practices and aim to avoid judging or interpreting them according to current standards (Allotey 2009). This chapter gives a brief snapshot of pre-twentieth-century birth attendance; a detailed examination of these events is comprehensively covered by Donnison (1988). Subsequent twentieth-century maternity policy and some poignant moments in midwifery and motherhood are summarised along with some key technological milestones. This is by necessity a taster, which requires the reader with whetted appetite to explore these issues in further detail (see Resources).

BIRTH BEFORE THE TWENTIETH CENTURY

Throughout the ages, the role of supporting women in childbirth has fallen to women, as part of their role as mothers and carers in close-knit communities. Indeed, up to the seventeenth century, the majority of midwives were women until the advent of the barber surgeon and the use of instruments and the obstetric forceps

(Kirkham 1996). Man-midwives, a term introduced into the *Oxford English Dictionary* in 1625 (Donnison 1988), began to be summoned for difficult cases as knowledge about anatomy was increasing and techniques were being introduced to facilitate birth. Prior to this and for centuries, women had always been cared for by women. Although most childbearing women continued to access the services of local women, being attended in birth by a male accoucheur was predominant practice with the upper classes by the mid-eighteenth century.

FAILURE TO PROGRESS

Obstetric practitioners of the period 1740–83, two Scotsmen, William Smellie and William Hunter, are heralded as contributing to great improvements in obstetric care, through education and training and refinements to the design of forceps (Drife 2002). However, it has been alleged that, in pursuit of knowledge and power to control and dominate this field, women were murdered to examine their anatomy, although there are no 'facts' to support this argument (Roberts et al. 2010). It is the case, however, that many women died in the 'man-midwifery' promoted lying in hospitals, from puerperal fever (Shelton 2012). Although the connection was beginning to be established that this infection spread between women, it was Hungarian physician Ignaz Semmelweis, director of the maternity clinic in Vienna in 1840s, who demonstrated that washing hands between undertaking post-mortems and attending women in labour could reduce their risk of contracting infection (Chamberlain 2006). Despite publishing a book on the subject, in 1861, his work went unheeded for many years and he was mocked by his medical colleagues.

SURGICAL INTERVENTION

It is probably a myth that the term 'caesarean' originates from Julius Caesar's mode of birth (Churchill 1997). It is more likely to have been derived from the Latin 'caedere', which means 'to cut' (Drife 2002). In Rome in 715 BC it became law, 'Lex Cesaria', that if a pregnant woman died, she should be delivered of the fetus so that they could be buried separately (Churchill 1997). The literature describing who first did what, how, where and when is contradictory. It is well documented that the caesarean was performed in many early civilisations, usually following the death of the woman (Newell 1921, Lurie & Glezerman 2003). There are reports of caesarean sections being performed in the sixteenth century on live women, but surgeons were divided regarding the virtue of the operation, which invariably resulted in the woman's death (Churchill 1997).

In Britain, during the mid-nineteenth century, the overriding concern of the majority of obstetricians was the safety of the mother in preference to the survival of the fetus. Hence until the possibility of maternal survival becoming more likely, destructive procedures such as craniotomy predominated for cases of obstructed labour. Before the introduction of chloroform by James Simpson in 1847, few women received any form of anaesthesia, although some operations were performed following intoxication with alcohol (Lurie & Glezerman 2003). It is likely that practices were introduced and developed subject to local culture, politics and decisions made by individual practitioners.

At this time, maternal mortality rates for caesarean birth in Britain were more than 80 per cent (Routh 1911), reflecting lack of experience, reluctance to intervene during early labour and poor antiseptic practices. In Europe, however, obstetricians began to embrace the concept of caesarean birth in favour of preserving life and delivering the fetus intact, probably strongly influenced by the doctrines of Catholicism, which predominated in these countries (Churchill 1997). Even in Europe, caesarean birth remained a highly hazardous procedure particularly for the mother, with more than half of women experiencing the procedure dying (Francome et al. 1993).

The male specialism continued to develop over the century as the value of the use of instruments in some difficult births was increasingly recognised. When the Medical (Registration) Act of 1858 came into being, requiring practitioners to gain medical credentials, women were excluded as they were prevented from being admitted to the medical register by the universities. Female midwives still practised but were seen as of lower rank to medical men working in institutions. However, many women did not want to be cared for by men and therefore did not seek the medical attention some might have needed (Donnison 1988).

Whilst the medical men were keen to keep a professional separation from midwifery practice, they had little inclination to attend long labours with little remuneration. They were generally in opposition to recognition of the midwife as a trained practitioner as there would be competition for their fee-paying patients. Poor women, however, could only afford the low fees of lay midwives and handy women (Kent 2000). In 1860, Nightingale set up a nurse training school in London, and whilst best known for her pioneering work in nursing, it was her aspiration to supply trained midwives to be able to provide a higher standard of care for rural women. However, the school closed in 1867 due to the number of cases of puerperal fever, and her dream went unrealised (Donnison 1988).

CATALYST FOR CHANGE

Midwives were fighting for registration in a political context where women had little power. Women were unable to vote, were often not financially independent and had little access to the education they craved. However, times were changing and women were demanding access to education on all levels.

The career of Elizabeth Garrett, who had paid high fees to undertake medical training and qualify as a doctor, was a notable point in history but it was not until 1876, ten years after her appointment as a medic, that women would be permitted entry to the British Medical Register. In the meantime, women were undertaking medical training and the 'Female Medical Society' was founded in London, with the intention of securing women's entry to the profession. Its college was run by Dr Edmunds, a consultant obstetrician, who was also an advocate of women's rights and follower of the principles of infection control proposed by Semmelweis. He was keen to separate midwifery from medical practice to spare women the indignity and health risks associated with male medical attendants; however, the college could only provide a few midwives a year and whilst welcomed by more affluent women, the poor were still attended by untrained midwives.

In 1870 an investigation into the high infant mortality rate (160 per 1,000 live births) was undertaken by the London Obstetric Society, which concluded that 70 per cent of births in England and Wales were attended by midwives, but that this varied depending on location.

Although opposed to the high-level training by the Female Medical Society, the Obstetric Society proposed prohibiting the practice of unqualified midwives and the setting up of an examination board to test their competence. With no movement from the government, the society set up its own exam board, with the requirement that the midwife should attend at least 25 labours but on certification would only be competent to attend natural births (Donnison 1988). Despite mixed critics of the proposals, the exam was set up in 1872.

THE MATRON'S AID

In 1880 a new midwifery society, 'The Matron's Aid', was founded by Louisa Hubbard, not a midwife but a supporter of women's rights for opportunity and employment (Donnison 1988). The society's aim was to recruit educated women as midwives, thus raising their status, further bolstered by the concept of having state registration. There was no intention to compete with the medical profession, instead their proposals were that the midwife's remit would be natural childbirth and that anything outside this remit would require the summoning of a doctor.

Members of the Matron's Aid were required to have the Obstetric Society's qualification, be 25 years of age or more and agree to follow an exacting set of rules. Their mission would be to promote health and propriety in their clients and ultimately save lives. Attempts to acquire support from the government for the registration of midwives hit many obstacles, however, including the fear that, if midwives were excluded from attending abnormal labours, they would be required to call a general practitioner who might not have any training in midwifery. Further, the Matron's Aid was few in numbers and did not represent the majority of midwives, hence progress was stilted. In 1886 there was a review of the medical profession which included that all future medical registrants would need to have a qualification in midwifery, as well as surgery and medicine, but it still did not make it illegal to practise midwifery or medicine without one.

THE MIDWIVES ACT 1902

Hansard (1892) records capture the moment when on 10 March 1892, a Mr Fell Pease asked Parliament to grant the setting up of a select committee to look into the issue of midwifery registration (HMSO 1892), which reported in 1893. However, it took eight subsequent attempts to introduce legislation before the historic Midwives Act of 1902 was eventually passed (Towler & Bramall 1986). This key moment in history set the president that it would be illegal for anyone other than a doctor or midwife to attend the birth of a woman, which is still UK law today. Local supervision of midwives was established to investigate poor practice and midwives had to report their intention to practise each year to the supervisory body in the area they intended to work; this requirement continued until March 2017. Whilst initially a predominantly punitive and regulatory process aimed at protecting the public from unsafe care, this statutory supervision also became a means of supporting midwives to develop and reflect. This provision has now been replaced with the non-statutory A-EQUIP (Advocating and Educating for Quality ImProvement) model (NHS England 2017), which is further discussed in Chapter 8.

EDUCATION FOR MIDWIVES

The 1902 Act also saw the creation of the Central Midwives Board, which kept a roll of all midwives and had the power to determine the training and examination requirements as well as the code of conduct to which all registrants had to adhere. To become a midwife, the training was initially 3 months, rising to 6 months by 1916, 12 months in 1926 and 2 years in 1938. There were shortened programmes for nurses and following the Committee on Nursing (1972) (Briggs Report), it became a prerequisite that all midwives should be nurses. In 1979, the Nurses, Midwives and Health Visitors Act established a new regulatory council, the UK Central Council (UKCC).

It was not until 1981 that a direct entry programme for midwives (3 years) was introduced and an 18-month programme for registered nurses to become midwives (Kent 2000). In the twenty-first century, 3-year programmes are the predominant means of qualifying as a midwife in the UK (see Chapter 4). The UKCC was subsequently replaced by the Nursing and Midwifery Council (NMC), which became the regulator for midwifery programmes in 2002 (Fraser et al. 2013).

THE LEGACY OF MIDWIFERY LEGISLATION

Despite the long gestation and difficult birth of the 1902 Midwives Act, it was not immediately implemented or adhered to. Many of the inspectors employed to investigate the quality of midwifery practice found that many midwives remained uncertified, and worked in unsanitary conditions, although this varied between cities (Dale & Fisher 2009). Subsequent Midwives Acts (1920) began to address the issue of midwifery representation on the CMB and required local authorities to provide maternity services (1936) (Kent 2000). It was the 1979 Nurses, Midwives and Health Visitors Act that amalgamated these professional groups for the first time, and a separate midwifery committee was established to ensure that midwives would not be overruled by the significantly larger body of nurses.

The autonomous practice of midwives as experts in uncomplicated maternities continued to be fiercely guarded and protected over the coming years. The Royal College of Midwives was named in 1947, emerging from its roots in the Matron's Aid Society. It continues to provide both a trade union and professional support to UK midwives (see Chapter 8) and defends the their role and sphere of practice, providing guidance and education to its members.

Changes to women's expectations and experiences of childbirth were influenced by the continuing emancipation of women, their role in the workplace and home as well as developments in technology. The following section considers some of the key advances in maternity care, beginning with the developing practice of caesarean section.

ADVANCING TECHNOLOGIES

CAESAREAN SECTION

Techniques continued to improve over the twentieth century with the advent of the transverse lower uterine segment incision, which healed faster than the classical incision and was less likely to become infected. This incision also led to the formation of a stronger scar than the classical method, with less likelihood of rupture during a subsequent pregnancy. However, this technique, although suggested at the turn of the century (Lurie & Glezerman 2003), was not widely adopted in Britain until introduced by Kerr (1926).

It is interesting that, despite increasing evidence that the new techniques were superior to the old, they were not adopted with haste. The method of incising the skin and fascia transversely was introduced by Pfannenstiel in 1900 and remains the method of choice today (Lurie & Glezerman 2003). This 'bikini line' incision is less painful than the classical incision and the subsequent scar is less conspicuous. Odent (2004) describes the introduction of the 'low segmental' technique in the 1950s in France. He suggests that it was slow to be adopted because obstetricians were reliant on their surgical colleagues for assistance and reluctant to compromise their own credibility and status.

Research into new practices continued to provide evidence of alternative, more effective techniques, including: non-closure of the subcutaneous tissue (Stark & Finkel 1994); blunt expansion of the uterine incision (Rodriguez et al. 1994); non-closure of the peritoneum (Irion et al. 1996); and double-layer uterine closure (NICE 2011). Caesarean section is now so prevalent in the UK at 30 per cent of all births (NHS Digital 2019) that it can be considered to be a relatively safe option by women, and some women request this option. NICE guidance is clear that women should receive information and counselling before such a request is granted, to ensure that the underlying reasons can be addressed and that the woman is aware of the relative risks compared with vaginal birth; these are outlined in the appendix to the guideline (NICE 2011).

Midwives have an important role in helping women to avoid unnecessary intervention. Whilst recognising that obstetric assistance can be life-saving, the impact of interventions that medicalise and reduce women's choices can have long-lasting impact on their emotional well-being (Schiller 2017).

PAIN RELIEF

The issue of pain relief in childbirth is complex; we know that the production of cortisol in response to stress and fear can prevent the release of oxytocin, hence potentially leading to delay and disruption to the progress of labour. In 1847, Queen Victoria is reported to have received chloroform during childbirth, administered by the obstetrician James Simpson (Bourke 2014). At the beginning of the twentieth century, the dubious practice of drug-induced 'twilight sleep' was introduced in some maternity hospitals whereby the mother would be anaesthetised, sometimes restrained, and wake up with no memory of the birth (Michaels 2018). The obstetrician Grantly Dick Read (1889–1959), however, is well known for his stance that childbirth was a natural process and that if women were properly prepared with knowledge and exercise they should have faith in their bodies to give birth without intervention. His book, *Childbirth without Fear* (Read 1944), provoked an interest in natural childbirth and the use of relaxation instead of the gas and air and other drugs that were also being introduced around the same time.

Yet the growing use of medical interventions in labour and the painful procedures that often accompanied them meant that there was a need for effective analgesia for women on the receiving end. The use of drugs that had been valuable during the First and Second World War were beginning to find their way into the labour room, such as trichloroethylene. Lobbyists, predominantly members of the National Birthday Trust Fund (NBTF 1945), campaigned to government to reduce maternal suffering and called for accessible pain relief for all birthing women (Caton 1996).

The use of pain relief in childbirth was debated in discussions about the development of the NHS, when in 1946 only 32 per cent of women had any pain relief in labour (Bourke 2014). The two sides of the debate, the right for women to have a pain-free birth and the availability of education and support for women who wanted to birth naturally, continued. Lamaze, a French obstetrician, published *Painless Childbirth* in 1956 based on what he learned from Russian psychologists on the art of 'psychoprophylaxis' using relaxation and deep breathing to cope with uterine contractions. Hypnobirthing is a current technique employed by some women, whereby they undertake an education programme and practise the techniques of self-hypnosis and relaxation during pregnancy with the aim of achieving a calm and drug-free birth (Mullan 2019).

NICE (2014) guidance for care of women in labour advocates that women should be supported in their choices for pain relief methods, including the use of water, breathing and relaxation, massage and the use of music. The use of pharmacological methods is also influenced by the woman's progress in labour and currently includes the availability of Entonox ('gas and air'), opioids, and epidural analgesia. There is growing recognition of the importance of the early connection between the mother and her baby at birth and the impact that drugs can have on this. Interestingly, the proportion of births where an anaesthetic or analgesic was given before or during birth has decreased from 67 per cent in 2008–9 to 61 per cent of births in 2018–19 (NHS Digital 2019).

OBSTETRIC PROGRESS

An interesting paper in the *British Medical Journal* written by Moir (1964) summarises the identification and use of ergometrine and Syntocinon, powerful uterine stimulants that have saved countless lives in the prevention and treatment of postpartum haemorrhage. The title of the paper, 'The Obstetrician Bids, and the Uterus Contracts', is apt, reflecting the power of the medical profession to intervene, control and influence the course of childbirth.

Whilst the prime aim of obstetricians has been to protect maternal and neonatal safety, sometimes the means were counter-productive in terms of the woman's experience. For example, in the 1970s the rising rate of induction of labour (IOL) was becoming a concern and led to an investigation by the NCT into the prevalence of the procedure, which was subsequently presented to the House of Commons (Kroll 1996). The use of IOL can lead to increased pain for women and therefore increased likelihood of her needing epidural analgesia. This in turn has led to an increased likelihood of her having an instrumental birth (pre-2005), although no increased risk of caesarean birth (Antonakou & Papoutsis 2016). A recent Cochrane review (2018) has concluded that, since 2005, the introduction of mobile epidural techniques has now reduced the associated risk of instrumental births (Anim-Somuah et al. 2018).

It is established, however, that IOL for pregnancies that are beyond 42 weeks gestation is associated with fewer neonatal deaths and fewer caesarean births than waiting for nature to take its course (Middleton et al. 2018).

FETAL MONITORING

Listening to the fetal heart during labour was undertaken on an intermittent basis using a Pinard stethoscope until the use of doppler ultrasound became available. The fetal heart was first detected electronically in 1906 and subsequently continuous electronic fetal monitoring (EFM) to facilitate variation and fluctuation in the fetal heart was first examined by Hon (1958). In the following decades the use of EFM became part of routine practice, despite lack of evidence to its efficacy.

During EFM the fetal heart is recorded simultaneously with the uterine contractions, via abdominal transducers attached by straps to the woman's abdomen, so that the baby's response to them can be considered clinically. Both wave patterns are recorded via a cardiotocograph (CTG) monitor either on paper or digitally. Its use, however, can restrict the movement of women in labour and require her to adopt a semi-recumbent position, which may impact on her experience of labour pain. Thus, systems have been developed to enable wireless EFM to facilitate active labour and birth, although this equipment is not universally available.

Programmes of education for obstetricians and midwives are mandatory to assist them in their interpretation of the CTG; however, they are open to considerable variation in interpretation. When there is a suspicious change seen in the fetal heart rate or variability, some practitioners often err on the side of caution and intervention to expedite the birth often follows. A Cochrane review (Alfirevic et al. 2017) concluded that there were fewer fits in babies who had been continuously monitored versus intermittently; however, there was no difference in the incidence of cerebral palsy. Continuous EFM is associated with an increased incidence of caesarean section and instrumental births and it is therefore recommended (NICE 2014) that low-risk women are not routinely monitored in this way. Further advances in the technology of EFM have led to the development of monitors that use a database of thousands of CTGs to analyse fetal well-being using a range of parameters, to help reduce misinterpretation and subsequent poor fetal outcomes (Redman & Moulden 2019).

ULTRASOUND IN PREGNANCY

Proposed as a tool to identify 'abdominal masses' by Ian Donald in 1958 (Donald et al. 1958), this technique of using ultrasonic waves to produce images has revolutionised modern obstetrics. The first fuzzy 2-dimentional pictures of the fetus have now been replaced by 3- and 4-dimentional images capable of identifying fine detail such as eye lashes and the anatomy of fetal organs. Initially used to estimate expected date of delivery, it is now employed for detailed fetal surveillance for all women at 20 weeks gestation and serially for women at risk of fetal growth restriction (for example, women who smoke) or with identified fetal compromise (for example, cardiac anomaly).

More recently it is recommended that all women have an estimated fetal weight measurement in addition to the anomaly screening at the 20-week scan and that women with high-risk pregnancies have uterine artery doppler measurements (NHS England 2019). The implications for training and scan capacity in many maternity units are considerable; however, the drive to reduce stillbirth and neonatal deaths is imperative.

FETAL MEDICINE

This is a branch of medicine that focuses on the diagnosis and management of high-risk pregnancies. Subsequent to the increasing ability for the identification of fetal disorders and complications, highly skilled obstetricians with additional training and experience in the field are able to monitor and manage the care of women to achieve an optimal outcome for the family. Many of the advances in the accuracy and resolution of modern ultrasonography has enabled specialists to diagnose congenital disorders in early pregnancy and in some case provide medical or surgical treatment in utero, to limit the damage to the fetus and increase its chances of a healthy life.

Such highly specialised services are only provided in large tertiary obstetric units where neonatal services are close by. Techniques include: intrauterine fetal blood transfusion (NHS 2019); in utero surgery for spina bifida (BBC News 2018); computer modelling of the fetal heart (BBC News 2019); and the radical technique of removing the baby from the womb, operating and then replacing it (Toyin 2019). Innovations continue to be developed which enable parents to make different choices about their babies' lives, where previously the options were termination of a pregnancy or the birth of a significantly handicapped baby. Now there are opportunities to monitor fetal development in order to optimise the right time and place of birth, so that a team of appropriately skilled surgeons and neonatologists can plan for timely treatment and care.

Despite the constant advances in technological support in childbirth, their availability, accessibility and acceptability vary, depending on where a woman lives and on her cultural and economic status. This is beautifully portrayed by Prue, who describes her contemporary work as a midwife in Australia and the diversity and dignity of the women she meets in her everyday practice:

> Women are goddesses. They are strong and they are courageous and I grow both personally and professionally with every encounter of which I'm given privilege. The Northern Territory of Australia brings together a multitude of diversity among age groups; cultures; ethnicities as well as socioeconomics; education standards and health complications.
>
> There's the young, pregnant Indigenous girl Careflighted [emergency air transport] in from her remote community having never laid eyes on a Caucasian; an elevator or even a sealed road. She should be home deciding on her after school activity or playing with her siblings but instead she is discussing her birthing options after a non-consensual conception. There's the couple who after years of trying to conceive with multiple unsuccessful IVF attempts are finally due to give birth to their first child and are overwhelmed by anxiety and fear. There's the middle-aged woman due to given birth to her 5th baby who is exhausted from her daily duties but so in love with the idea of number 5 and has a household of siblings dying to meet their new family member. Then there is the refugee who knows very little about the circumstances of her previous births in her home country. Some couldn't go home with her and she will never understand why. English is her second language and despite interpreters, she is terrified of medical staff and intervention because it is so different to anything she has encountered before yet all we want is for her to hold her perfect, healthy baby.

Nothing of course can prepare you for the loving mum who presents a few weeks out from her due date because she hasn't been feeling her baby moving and we have to deliver news of loss. We aren't taught how to handle so many situations but we learn on a daily basis how to support women and their families at times of vulnerability, of desperation, of devastation, of excitement, of exhaustion and of joy. Whether with a tear or a hug or some stern words of encouragement, the role of being an advocate allows me to empower women and for as long as they let me, I will continue to be part of their journey.

Prue Tierney, midwife, Australia

ASSISTED CONCEPTION

Since the birth of Louise Brown in 1978, the first 'test-tube' baby, there have been increasing developments it the field of assisted reproductive technology (ART). She was conceived by Invitro Fertilisation (IVF) whereby her mother's eggs were collected laparoscopically during a natural cycle, fertilised by her father's sperm in the laboratory and placed in her mother's uterine cavity at the eight-cell stage (Kamel 2013). Today the process of uniting the egg and sperm has many permutations, including: microsurgical epididymal sperm aspiration (MESA); *in vitro* maturation (IVM) of donor eggs; intracytoplasmic sperm injection (ICSI). Today, eggs are usually collected following hormonal stimulation; they are collected through a fine needle transvaginally and under ultrasound guidance. The availability of ART varies depending on where a woman lives, and the success rates also vary depending on the woman's age, health and reason for the infertility. Fertility treatment is closely controlled through legislation and monitored by the Human Fertilisation and Embryology Authority (HFEA).

SOCIAL AND POLICY HISTORY OF CHILDBIRTH

This section provides a summary of influential maternity policy in the last century. The extent to which this has been influenced by the power of the medical profession, advances in technology and the increasing volume of women's voices, including those of midwives, must be recognised. Increased availability and accessibility of research evidence to inform clinical maternity care was also key and was revolutionised by the publication of *A Guide to Effective Care in Pregnancy and Childbirth* by Enkin et al. (1989) and the establishment of the Cochrane Collaboration in 1993.

THE NATIONAL HEALTH SERVICE (NHS)

Created in 1948, this new NHS provision was a turning point for maternal and infant health. Now the attendance of a midwife, GP or consultant obstetrician did not incur a fee. Prior to its inception maternal mortality rates had been gradually rising between 1900 and 1937, when 1 in 250 pregnant women died. Following the universal provision of free health services for all, however, mortality rates were more closely scrutinised and started to drop. The system for reporting maternal deaths to a confidential enquiry was first introduced in 1952; prior to that they were reported to the Ministry of Health. The system on which it was based was created in 1928 in response to the high level of maternal mortality at the time (Snell 1928). Each confidential enquiry into a maternal death report covered a three-year period and followed a structured approach to examining the details of each death, collating trends and reporting on how care could be improved. However, it was not until the 1994–6 report that a midwife was included on the panel (Kee 2005).

PLACE OF BIRTH

At the turn of the twentieth century, childbirth was predominantly confined to the home with only 15 per cent of births in England and Wales taking place in hospital in 1927 (Loudon 2009). By 1932, births in hospital had already increased to 24 per cent. Childbirth was on the road to becoming safer with the use of oxytocic drugs and the discovery of sulphonamides to treat puerperal fever in 1937 (Smith et al. 2010). Midwives and General Practitioners (GPs) were still providing intrapartum care for many women at home. However, by 1965, 70 per cent of women were giving birth in an institution (Kroll 1996), meeting the aspiration of the Cranbrook Committee Report (1959). In 1970, the Peel Committee took the provision for hospital birth to its limits and decreed that all births should take place in hospital.

MEN IN THE BIRTH ROOM

Of increasing importance to women was the growing aspiration that their partner should be present at the birth. After the Second World War there was an increased emphasis on the importance of the mother–infant attachment on the emotional well-being of children (Bowlby 1953). This work was readily accepted politically as it coincided with the aspiration for men to regain their employment status, thus women were encouraged back out of the workforce, where they had made such an important contribution to the war effort, to resume their place as full-time carers. Subsequently, however, flaws in the underlying research were exposed and women began to campaign for better nursery provision (Thomson 2011).

However, in the late 1950s and 1960s men were already playing an increasing role in childcare, albeit predominantly as playmate (King 2012). Further fuelled by the increasing hospitalisation of childbirth in the 1960s and particularly after the Peel Report (1970), men were accompanying their wives and supporting them in the birthing room. Now a social expectation, being present at the birth of their child can be a life-changing event, as Stephen explains:

> As a father of three, now grown up children, my message is simple – be there at the birth.
>
> I accept that I was lucky in that all three births were relatively straightforward but the support we received from the midwives and medical staff generally made us feel we could have coped with most things. I say 'we' but of course I appreciate I was mostly observing and got to cuddle the baby after my wife had put in the hard work.
> It is a rollercoaster of a ride, and yes I did cry, but it is an event that will remain with me for the rest of my life, and there aren't that many things you can say that about.
>
> There was of course pain – but enough of the moment when my wife crushed my hand against the gas and air mask as she held onto me during a contraction! Seriously though, the arrival of your child is a momentous event. I want to pay tribute to the strength of character and courage shown by my wife. I will always remain utterly in awe of the way she coped with everything, and no, we boys couldn't!

> Being present at the birth is such a privilege and I believe has had a positive impact upon my subsequent relationships with my children. In my case it also undoubtedly strengthened my relationship with my wife. All in all, a pretty profound occasion.
>
> Stephen Swan, father and grandfather, UK

Whilst a positive experience can support a father's transition to parenthood, for some it is a source of anxiety, seeing their partner in pain and feeling powerless to intervene (Jomeen 2017). The midwife therefore has an important role in supporting birth partners to play an active role in caring for the labouring woman, and to recognise the long-term impact of the momentous events unfolding.

INFANT FEEDING PRACTICES

Breastmilk and breastfeeding are the optimal ways to nurture the newborn baby and developing infant. However, despite this knowledge, scientists have been endeavouring to develop an infant formula that could be close to breastmilk since 1865 (Stevens et al. 2009). This is an impossible task, as human milk contains so many bioactive properties that protect the infant from infection and inflammation, promotes healthy gut bacteria and growth and is unique to the age of the infant and even the time of the feed. Before the development of feeding bottles, use of animal milks and formula, 'wet nurses' were sometimes employed by the wealthy aristocracy to breastfeed their infants, and breastfeeding remained predominant in the working classes.

Over the past century, however, breastfeeding rates have declined from 90 per cent at the turn of the century, to 46.2 per cent at 6–8 weeks in 2018–19 (NHS Digital 2019). The proliferation of formula milk products and aggressive company marketing has sought to undermine women's confidence in the quality and accessibility of their milk. Despite the publication of the 'International Code of Marketing of Breast-milk Substitutes' (WHO 1981) the formula companies have found ways and means of promoting their 'follow-on' milks or 'specialist infant formulas' to meet and treat spurious needs.

However, those women and babies that do experience breastfeeding have the potential to experience a monumental connection, which is eloquently captured by Hazel, who remembers her feeding experiences of many decades ago:

> Breastfeeding at night is a gift. So beautiful. You lay in bed and can feel your breasts are warm and full with milk. You hear her snuffle in her crib, she doesn't need to cry. You talk to your baby and she will answer in her sweet baby talk. You pick your baby into your arms and she looks at you. You hold your beautiful baby close, close to you, close to baby. This beautiful baby will begin to drink your milk, you are together. We fall in love again.
>
> This is a special time. During the day everyone wants a piece of you, my darling baby, but now we are together just us two. In the morning your dad will say, 'another good night darling, she slept through again'. He will scoop you up in his big loving arms, and you will giggle together as you greet the new day. But we know.
>
> Hazel Walton, mother, UK

ESCALATING INTERVENTION

Oakley (2014) describes how in the late 1970s attention had moved from the impact of society on women's childbirth behaviours to the social, emotional and physical impact of obstetrical behaviour on women and babies. Disquiet about the overuse of interventions, the use of synthetic oxytocin to speed up labours and the indiscriminate use of episiotomy was voiced in the press, and debated by the medical and midwifery professions and general public. This led to the report to Parliament (DHSS 1977) highlighting the need for examination of the high rates of induction of labour, which had increased from 15 per cent in 1965 to 41 per cent in 1974 (Davis 2013). The public were also becoming more vocal about the escalation of obstetric interventions, which then led to further intervention; for example, induction of labour created more pain, which required epidural anaesthesia, which at the time also led to increased likelihood of instrumental or operative birth.

Concerns and exchanges about the impact of medicalisation and iatrogenic ill health (Illich 1976) in the general population became part of the commentary used by both user-led and maternity activist organisations. The work of the already established pressure groups – the Natural Childbirth Trust (1956) (which changed its name to the National Childbirth Trust in 1961 and is now known as NCT), the Association for Improvements in Maternity Care (AIMS 1960) and the formation of the Association of Radical Midwives (ARM) in 1976 – led to continuing pressure for services to reflect women's right to choose and be active partners in their birth experiences.

MALE MIDWIVES

It was in this time of increasing liberalism and the introduction of the Sex Discrimination Act 1975 (National Archives 1975) that men were also allowed to train as midwives in the UK. However, in contemporary maternity care, most midwives continue to be women; out of 36,914 midwives on the NMC register between March 2018 and 2019, only 106 (0.3 per cent) were male (NMC 2019); indeed 67 per cent of obstetricians in the UK are women (NHS Digital 2019). One male midwife talks about the sexism he has endured during his role and how often it is assumed that he is a doctor, which he has to manage carefully (Johnson 2019). One midwifery mentor described how she had anticipated there would be problems with women's partners when introducing her male student midwife to them, but found that men often welcomed another man in the room and found his presence a comfort to them (ARM 2000).

SHORT REPORT (SOCIAL SERVICES COMMITTEE 1980)

The reason for the enquiry which preceded this publication was purported to be public concern about the number of babies that were damaged or dying during pregnancy or following childbirth (Russell 1982). It called for better co-operation between paediatricians and obstetricians, that there should be more and better staffed neonatal intensive care provision. It was recommended that there should be better identification of mothers at risk and that antenatal care should be available in the communities where it was most needed to help reduce the numbers of babies that might be compromised at birth.

For the first time, it was suggested that women should be seen as partners not patients, their views should be sought and that care should be humanised.

WINTERTON REPORT (DEPARTMENT OF HEALTH 1992)

Labour MP Audrey Wise was distressed by the Short Report's focus on fetal outcomes and set up the Select Committee Enquiry, chaired by Nicolas Winterton, which examined the state of UK maternity services. This culminated in the publication of the Winterton Report in 1992 (Department of Health 1992), which promoted the values of woman-centred care and the increasing body of evidence that was being established through the work of organisations such as the National Perinatal Epidemiology Unit (NPEU) in 1977 and the publication of *A Guide to Effective Care in Pregnancy and Childbirth* (Enkin et al. 1989).

CHANGING CHILDBIRTH (DEPARTMENT OF HEALTH 1993)

This was a ground-breaking document outlining government policy for maternity services and built on the publication of the Winterton Report (Department of Health 1992). Chaired by Baroness Cumberledge, an expert maternity group was set up to bring together key stakeholders including the Association for Improvements in Maternity Services (AIMS), the National Childbirth Trust (NCT), midwives and obstetricians. A common vision was therefore created that had government support and reflected the voices of women as consumers and professionals. It outlined ambitions to provide care that offered choice, continuity and control to expectant mothers, delivered with kindness and shared decision-making.

This call to action led to the development of many initiatives in maternity services which recognised the importance of the woman's emotional safety as well as physical well-being (McIntosh & Hunter 2014). It was both an exciting and daunting time for midwives. Setting up and delivering services that provided antenatal, labour and postnatal care by midwives the woman had already met, needed considerable re-organisation and effective leadership. It required midwives to develop and maintain skills in all areas of maternity care, to offer home birth with confidence and provide a 24-hour on-call service, which often took them out of their comfort zone (Baston & Green 2002). Lack of funding and short-term implementation plan meant that many of the schemes Changing Childbirth generated were piecemeal or only sustained on the good will and enthusiasm of a few committed professionals.

THE NATIONAL SERVICE FRAMEWORK (NSF) (DEPARTMENT OF HEALTH 2004)

This strategy was built around the needs of the child and an aspiration to reduce the impact of the inequalities that many children are victims of. The socioeconomic and demographic differences associated with low breastfeeding rates, obesity, teenage pregnancy, substance misuse and chronic ill health prompted a targeted approach for families with low incomes. A schedule of contacts by key personnel was outlined and the importance of a smooth transition from midwifery to the health visiting service was highlighted as crucial to the accurate assessment of need for the child and family.

It heralded the advent of Children's Centres to provide support from conception to school age and hence as they emerged in communities, whereby many midwifery services migrated from health centres and general practices, into these shining, child-friendly venues. The Common Assessment Framework (CAF) was developed to identify the needs of vulnerable families in a way that was aimed to reduce duplication of effort and ensure that key agencies worked together to provide timely and effective support to protect and safeguard children. There was an emphasis on providing parenting information and support for parents from disadvantaged backgrounds.

MATERNITY MATTERS (DEPARTMENT OF HEALTH 2007)

Successive maternity policies built on each other's foundations. Continuity of carer remained a theme of Maternity Matters (2007) although with less emphasis on 'knowing the midwife' that supports intrapartum care, instead that 'Women and their partners will be supported by a midwife they know and trust before and after birth' (35). The element of choice was further developed highlighting that women should have choice regarding: how to access maternity care; what type of care they accessed; place of birth; and where to receive postnatal care.

It was envisaged that women would make an individual plan for care with their midwife or obstetrician discussing their care choices in relation to their specific needs and the provision of Children's Centres would be expanded from 1,000 to 3,500 by 2010. That midwives are the 'experts in normal pregnancy and birth' (15–16) was emphasised along with their role in providing a continuous link of support and coordination.

In recognition of the fact that women in disadvantaged groups had significantly higher rates of morbidity and mortality, this report placed significant emphasis on ensuring that maternity services were safe and provided by staff who were skilled and had access to continuous learning. This was against a backdrop of a reduction in junior doctors' hours and highlighted the need to provide flexible working and attract staff to enter, stay or return to clinical practice. It was hoped that getting the skill mix right at both ends of the workforce spectrum would release clinical time; for example, by employing consultant midwives and maternity support workers.

A national maternity data set was in development, so that outcomes between units could be compared against a robust set of metrics. In addition, satisfaction data would be collected from women to feed into continuous quality improvements.

Working towards a woman-focused model of care is not unique to the UK. In the Netherlands, for example, the model has long been based in primary care and provided by midwives; in 2005–7 the home birth rate was 29.4 per cent (KNOV 2017). Betty, a senior midwife in the Netherlands, describes her career through a time when midwifery-led care and collaborative working were key in the establishment of midwifery-led units:

> I worked for 20 years as a midwife in my own community practice with three other colleagues. We cared for approximately 400 women yearly during the prenatal, natal and the postnatal period. In 2007 ten midwifery practices started a midwife-led birth centre in the hospital nearby because home birth was declining and there was a need for a home-like environment with much focus on physiological birth. I decided to become the manager of that birth centre, because I really wanted to make this work. A personal factor to change jobs was that after 12 years of 24/7 responsibility I wanted a job in midwifery that would give me more time to pursue my other passion which is doing art.
>
> I worked for 12 years as the manager of this birth centre and I learned a lot! For example, how to improve the collaboration between all stakeholders' maternity care. It is quite the job to combine all the interests of community midwives, hospital-based midwives, obstetricians,

nurses, maternity care assistants, hospital staff and administration into safe and respectful care for women and babies. This was often a very political challenge.

Other challenges were to design a quality framework that was not only tailored to maternity care in hospital but also tailored to primary care. Or changing existing patterns of care into better ones. And all of that within creating a satisfactory work environment for care providers that were employed by the birth centre or worked closely with the birth centre.

Recently I moved to my next position of senior consultant in the national knowledge centre for maternity care assistants. A new challenge, now more nationally oriented. In this job I will continue to work on improvement of the system to ensure quality, safe and respectful care for women and their babies.

Betty de Vries, midwife, the Netherlands

Maternity care assistants are a valuable and well-established part of the maternity care team in the Netherlands and this is a model that units in the UK are beginning to embrace.

BETTER BIRTHS (NATIONAL MATERNITY REVIEW 2016)

Following extensive consultation with mother, fathers and maternity healthcare professionals and consumer groups, a new maternity strategy emerged from its long gestation. The vision was for women and their families to receive a kinder, safer and more compassionate service that met their personal needs and where they were informed and able to make decisions about their care. It published many recommendations, within seven key themes, which will now be described. It is current maternity policy in the UK, which all maternity units are working towards implementing.

PERSONALISED CARE

Women have access to information to inform their decisions through a digital maternity tool. They will develop personal pregnancy care plans, having chosen their care provider, and have a personal maternity budget through which to implement their choices.

The gold standard is that a woman should have continuity of care provided by a small team of four to six midwives that she has gotten to know during pregnancy and birth. There will be an identified obstetrician to work closely with each team.

WHY CONTINUITY IS IMPORTANT

When continuity is provided, the woman does not have to repeat herself to a new face each time she sees a midwife, but has the security of knowing that the team are aware of her health and social history and her birth experience. The midwives have a smaller caseload of around 40 currently pregnant women, and therefore have a detailed understanding of their needs; they also establish a rapport that supports communication and positive relationships. However, to provide care in a model where the number of midwives the woman encounters is limited to a pair or small team, means that ideally the midwives work full-time and take part in on-call or rostered labour ward night shifts. This pattern of working does not suit all midwives and does not account for situations where a woman might need specialist input or develops a condition during her pregnancy.

In a systematic review of randomised controlled trials, continuity of midwifery care was found to be associated with improved outcomes including increased likelihood of a spontaneous vaginal birth, less likely to have an instrumental birth and less likely to have a premature birth (Sandall et al. 2016). The review included 15 trials, published between 1989 and 2013 and involved 17,674 women from the United Kingdom (6) and Ireland (1), Australia (7) and Canada (1). The review often compared one team versus standard care and therefore its application across a whole maternity system was not tested.

Continuity of care is well liked by women and can give greater satisfaction to the midwives involved.

An Australian study involving 862 midwives showed that providing caseload midwifery contributed to higher levels of empowerment among the midwives and to lower levels of anxiety and depression (Fenwick et al. 2018). However, further research in needed to examine how it can be implemented for all maternity services, against increasing financial health service pressures and with an increasingly part-time midwifery workforce.

SAFER CARE

Maternity services should have a board-level safety champion who routinely monitors quality and safety, and these outcomes are used to compare performance with others and drive continuous improvement. Rapid referral protocols assist referral of women to specialists when needed. There will be a national investigation process to examine what happened when things go wrong, based in a culture of open and honest exchange with families.

BETTER POSTNATAL AND PERINATAL MENTAL HEALTH CARE

These services must be better resourced and services should be available for those who need care for longer, with a smooth transition between healthcare professionals.

MULTI-PROFESSIONAL WORKING

Based on the principle that 'those who work together should train together' both pre-registration and continuing professional development should embrace this standard. Nationally agreed indicators should inform what data is collected to reduce duplication of effort and these should inform the creation and use of an electronic maternity record.

WORKING ACROSS BOUNDARIES

Maternity service providers and commissioners should work together in local maternity systems (LMS) covering populations of up to 1.5 million. LMSs should come together in clinical networks to share outcomes and best practice.

A PAYMENT SYSTEM

Reform to current payment systems should create fair approaches whereby maternity units are appropriately compensated for the work they do and that money follows the woman and her baby.

WHERE ARE WE NOW?

In the UK, having gone through points in our history where women had few rights and pressure groups were needed to give voice to the plight of childbearing women, we are generally in a privileged position, where childbirth is relatively safe and the rhetoric of choice and personalised care resound.

It is important, however, to reflect on the plight of women around the world who are at very different points in their journey. As we heard in Chapter 1, providing midwifery care to all women would save thousands of lives, yet still so many women birth without the care and support of a skilled professional. The opposite side of the coin is the situation where women are bullied or coerced into birthing within a system that upholds the rights of the unborn child over their own right to choose, leading to court-ordered medical intervention and a culture of fear.

However, there is emerging hope as midwifery programmes are developing in areas of significant health need. For example, in 2013, professional midwives are being trained and introduced as practitioners in Bangladesh (Bogren et al. 2018). This is not without challenge, as the lack of respect for the profession by both the communities and medical colleagues, few resources and stressful working conditions frustrate the realities of becoming and being a midwife in the Bangladeshi health system and requires a cultural, political and economic shift to enable this work to progress.

There is a picture of struggle and hope in many other countries globally. For example, in Brazil, there are fewer midwives than there are in Sheffield, despite the huge number of births each year. However, the ICM Essential Competencies are now guiding midwifery training, with an emphasis on humanising the care of childbearing women (Gama et al. 2016). Inspirational midwives, like Natalia, passionately support the re-emergence and value of midwifery as a right that all women should have access to:

> Among many meanings of the word 'midwifery' in Portuguese my favourite is: to be with women. This definition expresses very well what it means to be a Brazilian midwife. Being a Brazilian midwife means facing many challenges. Brazil as a continental country encompasses multiple social and cultural contexts, with great diversity. In recent years we have advanced

in public policies for women's health, in 2005 the course of direct entry of midwives was reopened in the country, after the last class graduated in the 1970s. During this period different women filled the streets of some Brazilian cities to advocate for more rights at the time of childbirth. Being a midwife in Brazil is to stand up against a system that privileges and praises medical knowledge. It means fighting the inequalities that are marked by violence and maternal and child deaths, being a Brazilian midwife is striving incessantly for the guarantee of sexual and reproductive rights for all women of all ages and ethnicities. Being a Brazilian midwife is to see small scenarios change through good practice, to see women transforming their birth experiences into a cause, so that other women can live positive experiences too, enabling new lives to begin their trajectories full of respect and love. Being a Brazilian midwife is never giving up the small beginnings, is being with women for whatever comes united in community, because only then can change be possible. The voices of Brazilian midwives echo together: Brazil needs more midwives!

Natália Salim, midwife, Brazil

THE FUTURE

The Nursing and Midwifery Council (NMC) is responsible for the standards of proficiency for midwives and the pre-registration programme standards that student midwives must achieve in order to become registrants. Following extensive consultation with midwives, student midwives, academic midwives and women, these standards have been revised to reflect recent changes in demographics and the views and needs of women and their families. They are based on the International Confederation of Midwives (ICM) definition of a midwife and current best evidence and the quality framework presented in the *Lancet* series on midwifery (see Chapter 1). This comprehensive exercise was led by professors Mary Renfrew and Gwendolen Bradshaw; the standards were agreed by the NMC in October 2019, launched in 2020 and will be fully implemented by September 2021 (NMC 2019).

CONCLUSION

The development of midwifery and maternity care has taken many twists and turns throughout history. It has been influenced by a range of factors, not least the place of women in UK society and the subsequent value placed on women's health and related issues. The future destiny of midwifery depends on a continued recognition that the future well-being of society depends on babies having a good start in life and their parents being healthy and strong enough to support them in negotiating the path to maturity.

RESOURCES

Baby Milk Action, www.babymilkaction.org/about-us. As part of a global network campaigns and acts to protect breastfeeding and prevent deaths caused by formula milk marketing.

In vitro fertilisation (IVF): Human Fertilisation and Embryology Authority (HFEA), www.hfea.gov.uk/treatments/explore-all-treatments/in-vitro-fertilisation-ivf/.

Fox D (2011). Systematic reviews and health policy: the influence of a project on perinatal care since 1988. *Milbank Q.* 89(3):425–49, https://doi.org/10.1111/j.1468-0009.2011.00635.x. A useful review of the contribution of *Effective Care in Pregnancy and Childbirth*.

Gray M, Kitson-Reynolds E, and Cummins A (eds) (2019). *Starting life as a midwife.* Cham: Springer.

Hill M (2019). *Give birth like a feminist.* London: Harper Collins.

Kirkham M, and Perkins E (1997). *Reflections on midwifery.* London: Bailliere Tindall. An analysis of the issues that contribute to quality, woman-centred care, including the importance of choice, effective communication and social and cultural change.

Loudon I (1992). *Death in childbirth: an international study of maternal care and maternal mortality 1800–1950.* Oxford: Clarendon Press.

Oakley A (1984). *The captured womb: a history of the medical care of pregnant women.* Oxford: Basil Blackwell.

REFERENCES

Alfirevic Z, Gyte G ML, Cuthbert A, *et al.* (2017). Continuous cardiotocography (CTG) as a form of electronic fetal monitoring (EFM) for fetal assessment during labour. *Cochrane Database of Systematic Reviews* (2), doi:10.1002/14651858.CD006066.pub3.

Allotey J (2009). Writing midwives' history: problems and pitfalls. *Midwifery* 27(2):131–137.

Anim-Somuah M, Smyth RMD, Cyna AM, *et al.* (2018). Epidural versus non-epidural or no analgesia for pain management in labour. *Cochrane Database of Systematic Reviews* (5), doi:10.1002/14651858.CD000331.pub4.

Antonakou A, and Papoutsis D (2016). The effect of epidural analgesia on the delivery outcome of induced labour: a retrospective case series. *Obstetrics and Gynecology International*, doi:10.1155%2F2016%2F5740534.

ARM (Association of Radical Midwives) (2000). Male midwives, www.mid wifery.org.uk/articles/male-midwives/. Accessed 7 December 2019.

Baston HA, and Green JM (2002). Community midwives' role perceptions. *British Journal of Midwifery* 10(1):35–40.

BBC News (2018). Two unborn babies' spines repaired in womb in UK surgery first, www.bbc.co.uk/news/health-45958980. Accessed 3 December 2019.

BBC News (2019). Detailed images of baby heart inside the womb, www. bbc.co.uk/news/health-47638608. Accessed 3 December 2019.

Bogren M, Erlandsson K, Akter H, *et al.* (2018). What prevents midwifery quality care in Bangladesh? A focus group enquiry with midwifery students. *BMC Health Serv Res* 18, doi:10.1186/s12913-018-3447-5.

Bourke J (2014). The art of medicine: childbirth in the UK: suffering and citizenship before the 1950s. *The Lancet* 383:1288–1289.

Bowlby J (1953). *Child care and the growth of love*. London: Penguin Books.

Caton D (1996). Who said childbirth is natural? The medical mission of Grantly Dick-Read. *Anesthesiology* 84(4):955–964.

Chamberlain G (2006). British maternal mortality in the 19th and early 20th centuries. *J R Soc Med*. 99(11):559–563.

Churchill H (1997). *Caesarean birth: experience, practice and history*. Hale, Cheshire: Books for Midwives.

Committee on Nursing (1972). *Report of the Committee on Nursing (Briggs Report)*. London: HMSO.

Dale P, and Fisher K (2009). Implementing the 1902 Midwives Act: assessing problems, developing services and creating a new role for a variety of female practitioners. *Women's History Review* 18(3):427–452.

Davis A (2013). Choice, policy and practice in maternity care since 1948. *History & Policy*, www.historyandpolicy.org/policy-papers/papers/choice-policy-and-pra ctice-in-maternity-care-since-1948.

Department of Health (1992). *Health Committee Second Report: maternity services (Winterton Report)*. London: HMSO.

Department of Health (1993). *Report of the Expert Maternity Group: changing childbirth (Cumberledge Report)*. London: HMSO.

Department of Health (2004). National services framework for children, young people and maternity services, https://assets.publishing.service.gov. uk/government/uploads/system/uploads/attachment_data/file/199952/Na tional_Service_Framework_for_Children_Young_People_and_Maternity_Services_-_Core_Standards.pdf. Accessed 31 October 2019.

Department of Health (2007). *Maternity matters: choice, access and continuity of care in a safe service*. London: Department of Health, https://webarchive.nationalarchives.gov.uk/20130103004823/http://www.dh.gov.uk/en/Publicationsandstatistics/Publications/PublicationsPolicyAndGuidance/DH_073312. Accessed 24 August 2019.

DHSS (Department of Health and Social Security) (1977). *Prevention and health: reducing the risk*. London: HMSO.

Donald I, MacVicar J, and Brown T (1958). Investigation of abdominal masses by pulsed ultrasound. *The Lancet* 1:1188–1195.

Donnison J (1988). *Midwives and medical men*. 2nd ed. London: Heinemann.

Drife J (2002). The start of life: a history of obstetrics. *Postgrad Med J*. 78:311–315.

Enkin M, Keirse M, Neilson J, *et al.* (1989). *A guide to effective care in pregnancy and childbirth*. New York:Oxford University Press.

Fenwick J, Lubomski A, Creedy D, *et al.* (2018). Personal, professional and workplace factors that contribute to burnout in Australian midwives. *Journal of Advanced Nursing* 74(4): 852–863.

Francome C, Savage W, Churchill H, *et al.* (1993). *Caesarean birth in Britain*. Cambridge: Middlesex University.

Fraser DM, Avis M, Mallik M, *et al.* (2013). The MINT Project: an evaluation of the impact of midwife teachers on the outcomes of pre-registration midwifery education in the UK. *Midwifery* 29(1):86–94.

Gama S, Viellas E, Torres J, *et al.* (2016). Labor and birth care by nurse with midwifery skills in Brazil. *Reprod Health* 13, doi:10.1186/s12978-016-0236-7.

Hansard (1892). The registration of midwives, https://api.parliament.uk/historic-hansard/commons/1892/mar/10/the-registration-of-midwives#S4V0002P0_18920310_HOC_208.

HMSO (1892). *Report from the Select Committee on the registration of midwives*. London: House of Commons.

Hon E (1958). The electronic evaluation of the fetal heart rate. *American Journal of Obstetrics and Gynecology* 75(6):1215–1230.

Illich I (1976). *Limits to medicine: medical memesis: the expropriation of health*. London: Marion Boyars.

Irion O, Luzuy F, and Beguin F (1996). Nonclosure of the visceral and parietal peritoneum at caesarean section: a randomised controlled trial. *British Journal of Obstetrics and Gynaecology* 103(7):690–694.

Johnson S (2019). 'My tutor said it wasn't a job for a man': my journey from roofer to midwife. *The Guardian*, 9 May, www.theguardian.com/society/2019/may/09/tutor-not-job-man-roofer-male-midwife-nhs.

Jomeen J (2017). Fathers in the birth room: choice or coercion? Help or hindrance? *Journal of Reproductive and Infant Psychology* 35(4):321–323.

Kamel RM (2013). Assisted reproductive technology after the birth of Louise Brown. *J Reprod Infertil.* 14(3):96–109.

Kee W (2005). Confidential enquiries into maternal deaths: 50 years of closing the loop. *BJA: British Journal of Anaesthesia*, 94(4):413–416, https://doi.org/10.1093/bja/aei069.

Kent J (2000). *Social perspectives on pregnancy and childbirth for midwives, nurses and the caring professions.* Buckingham: The University of Buckingham Press.

Kerr J (1926). The technique of caesarean section with special reference to the lower uterine segment. *American Journal of Obstetrics and Gynecology* 12:729–734.

King L (2012). Hidden fathers? The significance of fatherhood in mid-twentieth-century Britain. *Contemporary British History* 26:25–46.

Kirkham M (1996). Professionalization past and present: with women or the powers that be? In *Midwifery care for the future: meeting the challenge* (ed. Kroll D). London: Bailliere Tindall.

KNOV (Royal Dutch Association of Midwives) (2017). Midwifery in the Netherlands 2017, www.europeanmidwives.com/upload/filemanager/content-galleries/members-map/knov.pdf. Accessed 6 December 2019.

Kroll D (ed) (1996). *Midwifery care for the future: meeting the challenge.* London: Bailliere Tindall.

Loudon I (2009). General practitioners and obstetrics: a brief history. *J R Soc Med.* 102(3): 88.

Lurie S, and Glezerman M (2003). The history of cesarean technique. *American Journal of Obstetrics and Gynecology* 189(6):1803–1806.

McIntosh T, and Hunter B (2014). Unfinished business: reflections on changing childbirth twenty years on. *Midwifery* 30(3):279–281.

Michaels P (2018). Childbirth and trauma, 1940s–1980s. *Journal of the History of Medicine and Allied Sciences* 73(1):52–72.

Middleton P, Shepherd E, and Crowther C (2018). Induction of labour for improving birth outcomes for women at or beyond term. *Cochrane Database of Systematic Reviews* (5), doi:10.1002/14651858.CD004945.pub4.

Moir J (1964). The obstetrician bids, and the uterus contracts. *BMJ* 2 (5416):1025–1029.

Mullan J (2019). What is hypnobirthing? www.hypnobirthing.co.uk. Accessed 7 December 2019.

National Archives (1975). Sex Discrimination Act 1975, www.legislation.gov.uk/ukpga/1975/65/enacted. Accessed 8 November 2019.

National Maternity Review (2016). Better births: improving outcomes of maternity services in England, www.england.nhs.uk/wp-content/uploads/2016/02/national-maternity-review-report.pdf.

NBTF (National Birthday Trust Fund) (1945). Newspaper article, *The Daily Mirror.* 69 H2/2, in: Caton, Donald. Who said childbirth is natural? The medical mission of Grantly Dick-Read. *Anesthesiology* 84(4):955–964.

Newell F (1921). *Cesarean section*. New York: D. Appleton and Company.

NICE (National Institute for Health and Clinical Excellence) (2011, updated 2019). Caesarean section CG132, www.nice.org.uk/guidance/cg132/chap ter/1-Guidance. Accessed 26 August 2019.

NICE (National Institute for Health and Clinical Excellence) (2014, updated 2017). Intrapartum care: care for healthy women and babies. NICE CG190, www.nice.org.uk/guidance/cg190. Accessed 3 January 2020.

NHS (2019). Blood transfusion to an unborn baby, www.nhs.uk/conditions/ rhesus-disease/treatment/. Accessed 3 December 2019.

NHS Digital (2019). NHS maternity statistics, https://digital.nhs.uk/data -and-information/publications/statistical/nhs-maternity-statistics/2018-19.

NHS England (2017). A-EQUIP: a model of clinical midwifery supervision, www.england.nhs.uk/wp-content/uploads/2017/04/a-equip-mid wifery-supervision-model.pdf. Accessed 4 November 2019.

NHS England (2019). Saving babies' lives. Version two. A care bundle for reducing perinatal mortality, www.england.nhs.uk/wp-content/uploads/ 2019/07/saving-babies-lives-care-bundle-version-two-v5.pdf.

NMC (Nursing and Midwifery Council) (2019). Standards of proficiency for midwives, www.nmc.org.uk/globalassets/sitedocuments/standards/standa rds-of-proficiency-for-midwives.pdf.

Oakley A (2014). The sociology of childbirth: an autobiographical journey through four decades of research. *Sociology of Health & Illness* 38(5):689–705.

Odent M (2004). *The caesarean*. London: Free Association Books.

Read G (1944). *Childbirth without fear*. New York: Harper Collins.

Redman C, and Moulden M (2019). Avoiding CTG misinterpretation: a review of the latest Dawes-Redman CTG analysis. *British Journal of Midwifery*, www. huntleigh.healthcare/_assets/img/PRODUCT%20PDF%20DOCUMENTS/ HUNTLEIGH-CTG-BJM-20140113101824.pdf. Accessed 7 December 2019.

Roberts A, Baskett T, and Calder A (2010). William Smellie and William Hunter: two great obstetricians and anatomists. *Journal of the Royal Society of Medicine* 103(5):205–206.

Rodriguez A, Porter K, and O'Brien W (1994). Blunt versus sharp expansion of the uterine incision in low-segment transverse cesarean section. *Am J Obstet Gynecol*. 171(4):1022–1025.

Routh A (1911). On caesarean section in the United Kingdom. *Journal of Obstetrics and Gynaecology of the British Empire* 19(1):1–55.

Russell J (1982). Perinatal mortality: the current debate. *Sociology of Health and Illness* 4(3):302–319.

Sandall J, Soltani H, Gates S, *et al.* (2016). Midwife-led continuity models versus other models of care for childbearing women. *Cochrane Database of Systematic Reviews* (4), doi:10.1002/14651858.CD004667.pub5.

Schiller R (2017). Birthrights comments on midwives and normal birth, www.birthrights.org.uk/2017/08/15/birthrights-comments-on-midwives-and-normal-birth/. Accessed 7 December 2019.

Shelton D (2012). Man-midwifery history: 1730–1930. *Journal of Obstetrics and Gynaecology* 32(8):718–723, doi:10.3109/01443615.2012.721031.

Social Services Committee (1980). *Perinatal and neonatal mortality. Second Report from the Social Services Committee 1979–1980 (Short Report)*. London: HMSO.

Smith A, Shakespeare J, and Dixon A (2010). The role of GPs in maternity care – what does the future hold? The King's Fund, www.kingsfund.org.uk/sites/default/files/Maternity.pdf. Accessed 7 December 2019.

Snell E (1928). Investigation of maternal mortality. *The Lancet* 211(5461):885–886, doi:10.1016/S0140-6736(00)97224-6.

Stark M, and Finkel A (1994). Comparison between the Joel-Cohen and Pfannenstiel incisions in cesarean section. *European Journal of Obstetrics and Gynecology and Reproductive Biology* 53(2):121–122.

Stevens E, Patrick T, and Pickler R (2009). A history of infant feeding. *J Perinat Educ.* 18(2):32–39.

Thomson M (2011). Bowlbyism and the post-war settlement, www.historyandpolicy.org/docs/thomson_bowlby.pdf. Accessed 2 December 2019.

Towler J, and Bramall J (1986). *Midwives in history and society*. London: Croom Helm.

Toyin O (2019). Baby operated on outside of womb for ground-breaking operation. *Independent*, 11 February, www.independent.co.uk/news/uk/home-news/baby-operation-womb-mother-spina-bifida-bethany-simpson-a8774081.html.

WHO (1981). International Code of Marketing of Breast-milk Substitutes, www.who.int/nutrition/publications/code_english.pdf.

BECOMING A MIDWIFE – A LEAP OF FAITH

INTRODUCTION

If you ask a group of midwives 'why did you come into midwifery?' there will be a range of responses as there are myriad reasons that draw people into the midwifery profession. For some it is the desire to work as an independent practitioner in a caring profession. Others may have been inspired by their midwife when they were pregnant or conversely by a determination to make a difference following a sub-optimal experience. Whatever the reason, taking the plunge, finding out more about the role of the midwife, what educational opportunities are available and what to consider when making university choices are important first steps. Completing an application and attending for interviews are the next steps along a career pathway that provides so much variety, job satisfaction and personal growth.

Each year, universities offering pre-registration midwifery programmes receive hundreds of applications from prospective students. In order to stand any chance of getting through to interview, it is essential that the application clearly demonstrates how the candidate meets the requirements of the programme and exceeds the requirements of the person specification. In this chapter we will explore what is on offer, and what it takes to succeed. But we will begin this journey with some philosophical considerations. This chapter is written for potential applicants and therefore addresses the reader as 'you'.

ART OR SCIENCE?

There has been much debate over the years regarding whether midwifery is predominantly an art or a science. Much of this discourse has been from an academic point of view; as you will see, pre-registration midwifery programmes differ in the qualification that is ultimately awarded, from Bachelor of Science (BSc) to Bachelor of Arts (BA). Ultimately, midwifery programmes will include elements of both natural and social sciences to ensure they prepare the student for holistic midwifery practice. At one end of the spectrum there lies the *positivist* dimension, which would suggest that contemporary midwifery should be based on knowledge derived from systematic review of the available evidence. At the other end is the *constructivist* dimension, which is supported by knowledge from intuition and experience (Power 2015). Before embarking on a midwifery career, it is important to consider the philosophy of midwifery and perhaps explore which end of the spectrum you favour or feel most comfortable with.

The simple answer to this conundrum is that midwifery is both an art and a science; they are not mutually exclusive. It encompasses the art of watchful waiting, listening, hearing and learning from observation that is passed from each generation of midwives to the next. Midwifery care is also based on the underlying principles of anatomy and physiology and a catalogue of scientific evidence which demonstrates one way of practising is better than another. Increasingly, qualitative evidence informs us how different approaches and models of care impact on those who provide and receive maternity services. Whilst we are autonomous practitioners, midwives always work within a social and humanistic context, we work with women and they influence and guide which approaches we take, depending on their specific expectations and aspirations. There is no 'one size fits all' approach to care. Midwives are encouraged as registrants to be reflective practitioners (NMC 2019a), to look back on our experiences and explore what happened and why, and then consider how we might do things differently in the future.

WHAT DOES IT TAKE TO BECOME A MIDWIFE?

INTRODUCTION

Applications to UK universities for pre-registration midwifery programmes are through UCAS (Universities and Colleges Admissions Service) and are made online before mid-January for that academic year. The process involves completing an application form, providing educational qualifications and employment history, a personal statement and providing the details of appropriate referees. There is also an administrative fee.

APPLICANT REQUIREMENTS

Applicants will normally be required to demonstrate they have a sound basic education, such as five GCSEs at grade C or above, including mathematics, English and a science subject. In addition, they will also need to have the equivalent of three A levels; access to higher education programmes are also considered. Work experience, especially in a caring environment, is a requirement of most programmes.

WRITING YOUR PERSONAL STATEMENT

The midwifery programme admissions team will be looking for individuals who have a sound understanding of the midwife's role. Therefore, it is wise that the applicant demonstrates they understand that midwives work in a range of settings and their work cover preconception to the postnatal period. Midwifery is multi-faceted and includes caring for women and their families from a diverse range of social, cultural and medical backgrounds, therefore the midwife needs to be able to work as part of a multi-professional team.

Applicants for midwifery programmes will usually have developed a range of skills during their life and work thus far that are transferable to the role of the student midwife. For example, a pupil who has worked as a waitress for a Saturday job will have learned interpersonal skills, by talking to members of the public and developing customer care approaches. They may have dealt with complaints and learned how to escalate difficult situations to their line manager. It is likely that during this work they will have worked as part of a team, looking out for new or junior staff and respecting senior team members for their experience and knowledge. It is important to show in your personal statement that you have considered what transferable skills you have developed and how they apply to the role of a student midwife.

We also learn transferable skills in unpaid roles, so it is also appropriate to outline, for example, how a role as a mother who juggles childcare and home-making responsibilities demonstrates the ability to manage competing priorities, problem solve and manage her time effectively.

HOW YOUR PERSONAL QUALITIES EQUIP YOU TO BE AN EFFECTIVE STUDENT MIDWIFE

Having excellent interpersonal skills and being a good listener are essential prerequisites for being a midwife. Pregnancy, labour and childbirth can be stressful situations and the midwife needs to instil calm in the mother, her partner and colleagues, at times of unpredictability and tension. Above all the midwife needs to be patient, to be confident to know when nature is taking the right course and facilitate space and peace to enable the woman to grow, birth and care for her baby.

Being able to provide examples of qualities that include taking responsibility for your own actions, whilst acknowledging the role of the wider team, is also recommended. The qualities of embracing diversity and respecting human rights are essential when working in the public sector with people who represent a range of religions, ethnicities and social backgrounds.

Having recent experience of higher education may be a requirement of the particular programme you are interested in. so, it may not be sufficient to have obtained an undergraduate degree 20 years ago, if you have not had any recent study demonstrating you are aware of the changing nature of the educational environment. Skills such as computer literacy and keyboard dexterity will be essential for success on a busy midwifery programme; having experience using online learning platforms, literature searching and email competence will be added bonuses.

WHAT NOT TO PUT IN YOUR PERSONAL STATEMENT

There is no need to have a witty opening line or a quote from literature, as these can detract from the essence of the statement, which should be about your motivation, appreciation of the role and your suitability to undertake it. It would be unwise to include in your personal statement that you want to be a nurse, which sometimes happens when a candidate has clearly cut and pasted a personal statement form a nursing application.

The personal statement should, above all, demonstrate that you have a clear understanding of what it means to be a midwife – 'having a love of babies' is not sufficient. Candidates sometimes make the error of only talking about the role of the midwife in relation to birth, rather than acknowledging the midwife's wider public health role in the antenatal and postnatal periods. Stating that you were inspired by TV dramas is also not ideal, as these are highly edited for entertainment purposes and do not always reflect the philosophy of contemporary, woman-centred care.

CHOOSING THE RIGHT PLACE FOR YOU

MIDWIFERY STANDARDS

All midwifery pre-registration programmes must meet the standards set by the Nursing and Midwifery Council to ensure that all midwives exit their education with the requisite skills and competence to practise safe and effective care. Following a comprehensive review of the evidence and a long period of consultation led by Professor Mary Renfrew (see Chapter 8), new proficiency standards have been approved and will be incorporated into midwifery programmes and fully implemented in 2021 (NMC 2019b). There are currently over 80 pre-registration midwifery programmes in the UK, so researching what is on offer is just as important as making sure you are an attractive prospective applicant. There are many aspects of the programme to consider in relation to your own personal philosophy and ensuring as good a match as possible from the information you can retrieve.

SPECIAL FEATURES OF THE MIDWIFERY PROGRAMME

All midwifery curricula must enable the student midwife to achieve the proficiencies (NMC 2019b), and the standards for pre-registration midwifery programmes have been revised to reflect these (NMC 2019c). However, each midwifery programme will have unique variations in emphasis. For example, some midwifery programmes are able to boast achievement of 'Baby Friendly' UNICEF (2019) accreditation, which means that they have undergone a rigorous assessment of their curriculum in relation to infant feeding and that this has increased the knowledge and understanding of their students. Other programmes have added extras, such as preparing students with the theory enabling them to undertake the additional skill of examination of the newborn. Some programmes include teaching additional, usually post-registration, skills, such as perineal suturing. The advantage of such programmes is that the midwife qualifies with the ability to provide this care to women rather than having to rely on another midwife to come in and undertake this function on her behalf. However, most maternity units have a programme of post-registration education (preceptorship) for newly qualified midwives that covers this, and much more.

Most midwifery programmes are undergraduate; however, some are now emerging at master's level, and therefore require advanced theoretical knowledge and application in practice. Another element to consider is if the programme you are interested in offers an elective placement and the opportunity to gain experience in another maternity unit in the UK or further afield. This can be incredibly eye opening, as there is a tendency to think that all maternity facilities function in the same way with similar philosophies and this is far from true.

Universities based in large cities will often offer 'home' placements based at the local maternity unit, and 'companion' or 'away' placements in localities further afield. The placement areas should be carefully considered in relation to the type and calibre of maternity units in which the midwifery students will gain their practice. Maternity units vary in terms of how many births they support, whether there are independent or alongside midwifery-led units or specialist fetal medicine and/or neonatal facilities. Health services are open to scrutiny by independent regulation (Care Quality Commission), based on a range of criteria, including: treating people with respect and involving them in their care; providing care treatment and support that meets people's needs; caring for people safely and protecting them from harm; staffing and quality and suitability of management. Full reports about individual maternity units are available online so that members of the public can consider these quality dimensions when they are selecting their place of birth. Trusts are also required to display their rating scores (outstanding, good, requires improvement or inadequate) where people can see them.

APPROACHES TO CURRICULUM DESIGN

Traditional undergraduate programmes often consist of a range of distinct modules that have independent assessments, run for a semester or two and then finish. Often a specific lecturer will be the lead for each module, perhaps with some invited speakers. Other programmes have a mix of short modules running concurrently with a longer, more practice-focused modules.

Approaches to midwifery education that use constructivist approaches encourage student-led discovery rather than directive teaching by experts (Patel et al. 2017). Some midwifery programmes use a problem-based learning (PBL) approach, which employs the use of trigger scenarios to prompts the students to identify what learning needs to take place in order to understand the situation. Tasks are then shared amongst the group and brought back for presentation at future sessions. Such approaches are useful to develop group working skills and to consider the complexities of physiology, pharmacology, sociology, ethics, etc. all together. This integrated approach enables students to understand how all the elements of knowledge contribute to the midwifery care we give.

Gilkison et al. (2016) describe the use of real-life narratives to enhance a midwifery curriculum in New Zealand. This involves a large class group listening to a narrative provided by either a woman, midwife or student. Similar to PBL, the group then subdivides to discuss what their learning themes will be, based on what the students determine are important issues raised by the real-life narrative. The topics raised are then supported by online material, clinical skills lab work, lectures and tutorials, as appropriate. Teachers support learning by facilitating group discussions, ensuring a safe environment is maintained so that all can share their views. The context of the narrative ensured that the importance of context is recognised: 'knowledge and skills are necessary for practice, but on their own are insufficient' (Gilkison et al. 2016:28).

THE UNIVERSITY

Aside from the actual curriculum and module line-up for a particular midwifery programme, it is also important to consider what else is on offer at a particular higher education institution. Things to consider might be student support and an active student union or post registration opportunities that might be available following the completion of this degree. It may be that there is an active research department with a well-recognised midwifery professor whose research you have been following. Whilst there are many universities that are well renowned for providing high-quality education or research opportunities to its students in general terms, the specifics of the midwifery programme should be considered as well as where the university falls in the overall league tables.

The campus location may be a relevant factor in making your choice. For example, some city universities have sprawling city-centre campuses and out-of-town complexes. Other universities are solely out of town and, whilst self-contained, may not suit someone who prefers easy access to city life.

THE LOCATION

This is another issue that is incredibly important when considering where to learn and develop your practice as a midwife. As already highlighted, many universities use a range of maternity units for student placements and this could therefore involve a significant amount of travel. It cannot always be guaranteed that a student will be placed nearest to where she lives. Although there will be a process for ensuring parity with other students across the length of the programme, being placed a long way from your accommodation in your first term, especially if you are moving away from home for the first time, can be challenging.

You may consider the distance from your hometown as a relevant factor in your choice. You may choose to commute or seek university or private accommodation, but it may be particularly important to be within easy reach of home if you have strong ties or particular commitments, such as ill or elderly relatives, for example. Moving away from home may also not be an option if you have children at school or because of your partner's work location. Alternatively, you may be free from such ties and wish to fly the nest and make a new start in a location far from home. In which case, you might consider a university based entirely on its strengths rather than contemplating its proximity to home.

If you have a particular interest that you wish to explore in the time that you are not studying or on placement, the location can also be a key factor in the decision. For example, you may enjoy cycling or rock climbing and look for a city that has easy access to locations where you can enjoy these sports. You may have an interest in live music and want to be close to a vibrant rock venue that attracts a particular genre. You may crave easy access to a beach or to a city if you come from a small town – the options are endless and there is a study location to suit most needs.

OPEN DAYS

It is essential that you check out the course, university and location for yourself. These can be booked directly with the university you are interested in and information is also available on the UCAS website. You will find out so much more by experiencing what it feels like to walk around a campus and meet other students, away from the rhetoric of carefully crafted programme web pages. Take someone with you who can see things from a different perspective and help you reflect on what you hear and see. It is a lot to take in and can be an expensive trip, but it's worth experiencing the reality to help inform your decision.

MAKING THE DECISION

Not all of the criteria we have discussed will have the same weight for each person. Ultimately, the decision regarding where to study midwifery may come from a gut reaction following attending an open day or may be the results of a structured analysis of the pros and cons of each of your short-listed options. Whichever method you use to reach a conclusion, it is always wise to talk things through with someone you trust. Articulating how you feel and what your impressions are will help you to formulate your ideas. There are some useful tools to help with the process, depending on your own particular style, for example, provided by Health Education England (HEE 2019).

MAKING THE GRADE

THE INTERVIEW PROCESS

Many universities hold a selection process that spans a whole day. It may start with an overview of the programme by members of the lecturing team, followed by group activities and then individual interviews. Some universities require the applicant to undertake a short written piece of work on the day, not necessarily to test knowledge but to provide information about their ability to construct an argument and articulate their thoughts. Universities are accustomed to making suitable adjustments for students with dyslexia and dyspraxia and these challenges can be accounted for. It is common for the selection process to include experienced midwives and also service users, so that candidates with genuine caring and compassionate potential can be identified.

During group activities, where a small group of candidates are asked to discuss a topical issue, the panel are looking for candidates who can demonstrate the ability to join in and offer constructive suggestions to the challenge. They also want to observe candidates being respectful of others and who are not trying to monopolise the conversation. This can take individuals out of their comfort zone, but it is important to contribute to the activity, even if you agree with everything that is being raised and cannot think of a new alternative.

BEING OFFERED A PLACE

If successful in being offered a university place, applicants must agree to having a police check, known as a DBS check (Disclosure and Barring Service), to demonstrate that they have no current criminal convictions. This check is carried out at the highest 'enhanced' level because the student midwife will be working with vulnerable adults and children and will therefore be screened for previous offenses including: sexual, violence, the supply of drugs and safeguarding. DBS checks are usually renewed every three years although a registrant is required to notify their employer if they are convicted of an offence in the intervening period.

Being offered a place on a midwifery programme is a real achievement; there are so many applicants for relatively few places so getting this far is great news. However, the hard work starts here and there are many things to consider that will be helpful to achieve success.

STAYING THE COURSE – SINK OR SWIM?

STUDY SKILLS

Being a student midwife is hard work. It requires determination and dedication as well as academic ability. Having tried-and-tested study skills will be invaluable as the student midwife has to learn to juggle competing priorities. Not everyone learns in the same way: some prefer to see things visually, using mind maps and colours to help them remember key facts; others use summarising techniques, reading a text and then making notes. Take advantage of the study skills sessions that are available for new students – it may be that the best way for you to learn is yet to be encountered.

Getting feedback about your academic performance is particularly useful, so that you understand the required level of research and that you feel confident you are getting the essay-writing technique up to scratch. Most programmes encourage you to seek academic support either from your personal tutor or the module leader; either way, take advantage of their precious time and ensure you seek timely help rather than leaving it to the last minute. If you have not pitched the assignment at the right academic or content level, there will be little time to make amendments if you ask for help close to the deadline.

PRACTICE TIME

Learning to be a midwife involves both theoretical study and clinical practice and therefore the responsibility to provide relevant and coherent learning opportunities is shared equally between the university lecturing staff and clinical midwives. The student midwife will usually work in a range of practice settings throughout their education programme that are likely to involve significant travelling, sometimes on dark cold mornings to get to work for an early shift or going to work in the evening when other students are getting ready to go to the bar. Every day in practice is accounted for, therefore if the student misses placement time due to ill health or compassionate leave, they will need to make that time up. And as if that is not challenging enough, they will also be writing and submitting academic work throughout their programme so they will need to be extremely disciplined and organised to ensure that they meet all the necessary deadlines.

DEVELOPING CLINICAL SKILLS

There are many fantastic simulation aids that are used in contemporary midwifery undergraduate programmes. Some universities have invested in state-of-the-art simulation laboratories; indeed, that may have been the particular feature that helped you make your choice. Simulation is valuable for students to learn together in a safe environment. Standing around a bed with a manikin to practise abdominal palpation enables students to learn from each other, to make light of issues they do not understand and to practise the same technique repeatedly. Clearly it would not be appropriate for a gang of student midwives to do this with real pregnant women (although it was a model of practice for many medical students in previous years).

Simulation is no replacement for the real thing and caring for women; therefore, the best way to learn the art and science of midwifery is working alongside a clinical midwife who can provide mentorship and supervision whilst caring for women and their families. Real women will tell their individual stories and contextualise the skill that the student is trying to learn. So, for example, a student might find it difficult to find a fetal heart during an antenatal assessment. A woman can provide helpful hints, such as 'her back is at this side', or 'they usually find her heartbeat just here'. Thus, the student learns from partnerships between midwives and women, applying theoretical knowledge in the practice setting.

SURVIVAL OF THE FITTEST?

We have already advised that becoming a midwife, learning the skills and gaining the required competencies takes time. It is impossible for students not to compare themselves with others on the same programme and listen to their peers describe the various opportunities that they have had. Some experiences do not present themselves very often; for example, witnessing a twin or vaginal breech birth. Others might be dependent on working in a particular team of midwives; for example, a home birth or continuity team. Ultimately, student midwives all have to achieve the minimum standards to register as a midwife, but the range of experiences each individual student has been exposed to will vary.

THE ROLE OF THE CLINICAL MENTOR

The generic term 'mentor' is used in the context of this book to describe a midwife who provides a role model and supports learning in the clinical setting. However, there are a range of terms used to describe the distinct roles and responsibilities of a range of registrants who guide, supervise and assess students and these include 'practice supervisors', 'practice assessors' and 'academic assessors' (NMC 2018b). When student midwives are on clinical placements they are assigned to work with an experienced midwife who will be responsible for ensuring that the student is supervised and has some continuity of support and mentorship so that progression, or lack of it, can be identified. It takes time to get to know each other and spending a lot of time in close proximity can be difficult at times. Most importantly, it is wise not to make assumptions, for example, that a mentor who is quiet does not like you, or that a midwife who is chatty wants to be your best friend. The relationship should remain professional at all times and one where each party feels that they can be honest about how they are feeling whilst respecting each other's positions.

SUPERVISION

It is usual for a mentor to want to ensure that she is confident that the student can undertake an aspect of clinical care with skills and accuracy before she allows the student to work independently with some tasks. The student midwife should expect this and not be disheartened if she had learned how to do blood pressures with one mentor and then the next one is checking that she is competent again. The mentor responsible for a student can only delegate tasks that the person is capable of doing: she will ultimately be responsible if a student makes a mistake, so confirming competence is usual practice.

SUPPORTING THE MENTORS

Midwives who mentor pre-registration students also need preparation and support. High levels of activity in maternity units mean that mentors need to develop trusted techniques for ensuring they provide adequate supervision and effective coaching, whilst continuing to provide personalised care to women (Cummins et al. 2013). The NMC (2018a) have issued Standards for Education and Training, which include: a framework for promoting a learning culture; ensuring quality and compliance with legal requirements; empowering students; preparation of educators and assessors; and setting standards for curricula assessments. It outlines that those who support students in practice must have adequate induction to their role and be supported by time and resources to fulfil their responsibilities. Student assessment must avoid subjectivity and should therefore be based on evidence of student performance.

To ensure that assessment of student proficiency is robust and evidence based, the NMC requires students to be assigned to a nominated practice assessor who is a registered midwife, for clinical placements (NMC 2018b).

SINK OR SWIM?

LOOKING AFTER YOURSELF

Becoming a student midwife is a hugely exciting but often daunting journey to begin and the path may not always be smooth. Whilst you can consider all of the issues already discussed above, there will be events that occur without warning and that could not have been anticipated. Of course, life throws up many such issues and just because you are a student midwife does not mean that you will be more prone to these; however, the emotional road thus travelled – applying, choosing, interviews, acceptance – means that there may be considerable weight on your shoulders to succeed, having got this far.

University staff, however, are used to helping students with life's challenges and it is important that you communicate with your lecturers, perhaps personal tutor or year leader, if something happens that derails you. They might not be able to intervene or orchestrate a solution themselves, but they will be able to point you in the right direction of identifying someone who can provide confidential support whether that is financial, educational, health or emotional from someone you can trust. Sometimes it becomes necessary to take time out, and this can usually be facilitated but might mean that the most appropriate option is to take a whole year out.

Lecturers in midwifery have all been practising midwives. They know what it is like to feel vulnerable and uncertain at times. They have chosen the path of education to support and care for students, as Sally clearly demonstrates:

> I have always felt incredibly proud and privileged to be a midwife, but to me, being a midwifery lecturer is an absolute honour. I marvel every day that I have a job where I can advise, influence and educate the midwives of the future. I practised for 25 years as a midwife before becoming a lecturer, and I feel that being a lecturer is similar to being a community midwife, with my caseload being my students. I love being able to advise, signpost and guide students until they grasp a concept. I clearly recall not being able to understand aspects of anatomy and physiology, and I think this helps with trying to use different methods to aid understanding. I encourage my students to take note of the world around them; to take an interest in politics and feminist issues, so they can represent all women and not just pregnant and newly birthed women.
>
> Being resilient is a really important part of being a midwife, and so when students need to discuss a difficult shift, or a personal issue, I feel that an essential thing I do is to find time to speak with students, and to sometimes help to put things into perspective with them. A chat and a bit of one to one time, goes a long way.

My favourite part of all is being a role model for my students. The most important thing a midwife needs to be is kind, and I try to instil this in all students from day one. To have knowledge, patience and inquisitiveness is important, but to have the simple trait of being kind, is crucial to being 'with woman' – a midwife. This is what women will always remember you for.

Sally Freeman, senior midwifery lecturer, UK

QUALIFYING AS A MIDWIFE

PRECEPTORSHIP

Qualifying as a midwife is a rite of passage, but the learning continues and working as an independent practitioner and making your own decisions can be daunting. However, most maternity units will have a detailed and structured preceptorship package, during which time the preceptee learns how things are done in that particular organisation. There will be some supernumerary time, although this will vary from unit to unit, while the midwife awaits her NMC registration number, gets her uniform and security badges, etc. There will be a Trust induction as well as induction to the maternity unit, and it may seem as though there is a lot of information that does not feel relevant to the role of the midwife. However, it is important to engage with the opportunities that are available in the wider Trust and that the midwife learns about the other roles that will support her care giving.

During the preceptorship period, the newly qualified midwife will be supported to continue to consolidate their pre-registration learning whilst gaining the additional skills required to provide holistic care to women. This support will be in partnership with a nominated preceptor and often with the support of the clinical educators (see Chapter 8). Accomplishing a prescribed list of skills, including epidural top-ups, intravenous drug therapy and perineal suturing, will be part of the preceptorship package and success in its completion is often accompanied with eligibility to progress to the next clinical grade.

REVALIDATION

Continuous learning is a prerequisite of maintaining professional registration. This currently involves fulfilling a range of criteria, including:

reflecting on practice; having reflective discussions with another registrant; undertaking at least 450 practice hours every three years; undertaking 35 hours of continuous professional development; and self-declaring good health and character (NMC 2019a). The midwife also needs to provide five pieces of practice-related feedback. All of the above must be signed off by a 'confirmer', usually the midwife's line manager. The process is designed to support midwives to learn from their experience and educational opportunities, to seek feedback and to discuss and reflect on clinical care.

CONCLUSION

The journey to becoming a midwife requires considerable personal investment and determination. There are a range of elements to consider; not just what educational institutions can offer you, but how your skills, experience and personality match the requirements of the programme and the profession. Where you ultimately begin your studies as a midwife will depend on a range of factors — where you end up is up to you. The sky's the limit!

RESOURCES

Care Quality Commission (CQC), www.cqc.org.uk/. This website provides information about the criteria that are used to assess the quality of a healthcare environment and the facilities and staff that are available. Full inspection reports are available about individual units.

League tables for universities, www.thecompleteuniversityguide. co.uk/league-tables/. This useful website also hosts information about different courses, fees and open days, searchable by subject and location.

Royal College of Midwives (RCM). How to become a midwife, www.rcm.org.uk/promoting/learning-careers/become-a-midwife/. This resource combines videos and Q&A responses to assist those thinking of a career in midwifery. It also contains information about the range of settings in which a midwife works, and expected pay and conditions.

UCAS (Universities and Colleges Admissions Service), www.ucas. com/ucas/after-gcses/find-career-ideas/explore-jobs/job-profile/mid wife. This is an excellent source of information for prospective students, not just about courses and how to apply for them but also student finances, careers advice and student well-being. Application deadlines, www.ucas.com/advisers/managing-applications/application-deadlines.

REFERENCES

Cummins A, Catling C, Hogan R, *et al.* (2013). The art and science of supporting midwifery students in clinical practice. *Women and Birth* 26(1):S42–S43.

Gilkison A, Giddings L, and Smythe L (2016). Real-life narratives enhance learning about the 'art and science' of midwifery practice. *Advances in Health Sciences Education* 21(1):19–32.

HEE (Health Education England) (2019). Health careers. Decision making. Career planning, www.healthcareers.nhs.uk/career-planning/improving-your-chances/planning-your-career/decision-making. Accessed 12 October 2019.

NMC (Nursing and Midwifery Council) (2018a). Realising professionalism: standards for education and training. Part 1: standards framework for nursing and midwifery education, www.nmc.org.uk/globalassets/sitedocuments/education-standards/education-framework.pdf. Accessed 12 October 2019.

NMC (Nursing and Midwifery Council) (2018b). Realising professionalism: standards for education and training. Part 2: standards for student supervision and assessment, www.nmc.org.uk/globalassets/sitedocuments/education-standards/student-supervision-assessment.pdf. Accessed 12 October 2019.

NMC (Nursing and Midwifery Council) (2019a). Revalidation. Your step-by-step guide through the process, http://revalidation.nmc.org.uk. Accessed 12 October 2019.

NMC (Nursing and Midwifery Council) (2019b). Standards of proficiency for midwives, www.nmc.org.uk/globalassets/sitedocuments/standards/standards-of-proficiency-for-midwives.pdf. Accessed 12 October 2019.

NMC (Nursing and Midwifery Council) (2019c). Standards for pre-registration midwifery programmes, www.nmc.org.uk/globalassets/sitedocuments/standards/standards-for-pre-registration-midwifery-programmes.pdf. Accessed 12 October 2019.

Patel S, Wallis-Redworth M, Jackson S, *et al.* (2017). Art and science: promoting understanding and empathy through film. *British Journal of Midwifery* 25(11):734–740.

Power A (2015). Contemporary midwifery practice: art, science or both? *British Journal of Midwifery* 23(9):654–657.

UNICEF (2019). Guide to the UNICEF UK baby friendly initiative university standards. Baby friendly standards. Standards for universities, www.unicef.org.uk/babyfriendly/wp-content/uploads/sites/2/2019/07/Guide-to-the-Unicef-UK-Baby-Friendly-Initiative-University-Standards.pdf. Accessed 20 October 2019.

5

PRE-CONCEPTUAL AND ANTENATAL CARE

INTRODUCTION

Pregnancy is a time for women to reflect on their bodies and how they can best prepare for the important role of nurturing new life. It can provide the impetus for making significant lifestyle changes, for turning away from the freedom and self-centred nature of early adulthood and taking responsibility for the environment in which their baby will develop and grow. However, this utopian aspiration is far from reality: many women are approaching motherhood later in life with deep-rooted habits, routines and practices or with an underlying medical condition. They may already have health challenges that need to be considered by the midwife when planning pre-conceptual and antenatal care. This chapter will look at the ways that midwives can influence the health of women and babies before conception and during pregnancy. It begins with an overview of the midwife's role in antenatal care using the patchwork model (see Figure 5.1) described in Chapter 2.

PROFESSIONAL – ACCOUNTABLE AND SAFE

A professional is someone who is skilled, proficient and qualified. However, behaving in a professional manner requires the midwife to be courteous, attentive and generate confidence, so that women feel in safe hands. Appearances can be deceptive and whilst at one time in history nurses and midwives had to look the part and wear American tan tights and a stiffly starched cap, behaving professionally is so much more than that. Midwives come in all shapes

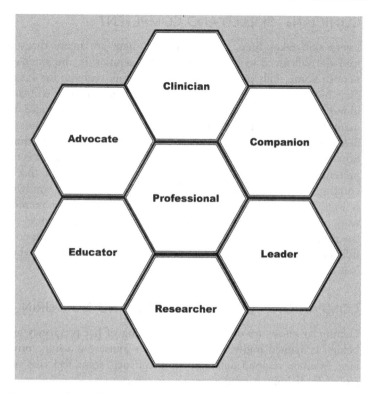

Figure 5.1 The midwife's role: patchwork model

and sizes, exercising their personality through a variety of hair colours and skin art. However, it is the midwife's demeanour and compassion that will influence the woman's perception of her professionalism.

Pregnancy may be the first time that a woman has set foot inside a hospital. She may have preconceived ideas about what will happen to her. Whilst her expectations may be influenced by the media and what she has heard from friends and family, how she perceives that experience will be personal to her and defined by how she is greeted, treated and cared for by the staff she meets. The manner in which care is given is crucial, including the tone and inflection of the voice and non-verbal behaviour.

CLINICIAN – SKILLED AND COMPETENT

Every skill takes time to develop and there are many that the midwife will need to acquire to care for women in the antenatal period. Some skills are generic to caring for all women; for example, the midwife will need to be proficient in taking a woman's blood pressure, pulse and testing her urine. However, there are many that are unique to the midwife's role, hence they cannot be delegated to a nurse or healthcare assistant. For example, learning how to palpate a woman's abdomen in order to detect what is the presenting part (whether it is the fetal head or bottom that is coming first) takes practice. Gradually the student midwife is introduced to this art as she observes her midwifery mentor, reads about the technique in midwifery texts and then applies the theory to practice. Eventually she will perform this skill with confidence and competence, although there will always be times when it is difficult to discern the fetal position.

COMPANION – COMMUNICATING AND NURTURING

Getting to know a woman at the beginning of her pregnancy and being her named midwife throughout her journey is a huge privilege. Women respond differently to pregnancy, some feel very sick and overwhelmingly tired, especially in the first trimester. Others do not appear to be any different and bloom from the start. However, pregnancy can leave a woman feeling vulnerable and out of control as her body changes and grows in ways that she has little power to influence. Emotions run high and the support of a kind and experienced midwife can be reassuring and empowering. Women need feedback about their health and progress throughout pregnancy. The midwife needs to be able to convey important results or even simply take the time to inform the woman of routine measurements such as what her blood pressure is and what it means.

ADVOCATE – PROTECTING AND ENABLING

There are times when women need additional support from their midwife, perhaps if they have an aspiration to do something that is not usually part of traditional care. Perhaps a woman had a particularly traumatic birth in her first pregnancy and now wants to give birth without technology despite a previous emergency caesarean. The woman should not have to feel that she is 'fighting the system' but that someone has her best interests at heart. The midwife will need to acknowledge how the woman feels and aim to find a solution that is both safe and facilitates the woman's needs. This may mean that she supports the woman when she attends for a consultant appointment or suggests a plan of care that provides a midwife-led approach, but with obstetric support on hand.

EDUCATOR – FACILITATING LEARNING

Each woman will start her pregnancy with a different level of knowledge regarding what the future holds in store. Some will have done a significant amount of research on the internet before getting pregnant and others will not necessarily have planned their pregnancy and have limited knowledge about their options, what will happen to their body or how to find out more. The midwife will be an important point of information as well as the person who can signpost to other authoritative sources. The midwife also has a role in correcting myths and misinformation, to ensure that the woman has access to the facts to enable her to make appropriate choices. In order to personalise care, the midwife should always start out with, 'What do you know about …?' so that she can fill in any gaps.

Not all women want or are ready to receive information and this will vary depending on the stage of their pregnancy. For example, at the booking appointment the woman may not be able to see past having her first scan, and will not therefore want to talk about feeding her baby. The midwife therefore needs to pitch her information giving to the woman's personal needs.

RESEARCHER – CREATOR OF NEW KNOWLEDGE

Knowledge is constantly evolving and the midwife needs to keep abreast of new evidence and be able to disseminate it to both her colleagues and women on her caseload (NMC 2019). It should never be assumed that because a woman has had a baby before she is aware of the most recent information. Advice changes as new knowledge develops; for example, it has recently been confirmed that the sleeping position of pregnant women in the antenatal period can influence their chances of having a stillbirth (Heazall et al. 2017). The Midlands and North of England Stillbirth Study (MINESS) compared the sleeping position of women who had a stillbirth with case controls who had not. It found that women who went to sleep on their side in the last trimester of pregnancy were less likely to have a still birth than woman who went to sleep on their backs, with an estimated saving of around 130 babies per year. This information therefore needs disseminating to all women so that they can adapt their sleep practices accordingly. Women should be reassured that it is being on their side when they go to sleep that matters and not to worry if they change position in the night, but to turn on to their side again to resume their sleep if they wake.

LEADER – CHANGE AGENT

Midwives caring for a caseload of women in the antenatal period need support and guidance. There will often be challenges when a situation arises that has not previously been encountered. Having supportive leadership is key to enabling midwives to flourish and develop as they learn from experience and that of their colleagues. Having reflective time together as a team can be an invaluable means of sharing ideas and challenges, where concerns can be raised in a non-judgemental forum. Leadership can be evident at all levels of seniority; having the determination to provide excellent care will empower even the most junior midwife to speak up and challenge inappropriate practice.

PRE-CONCEPTUAL AND ANTENATAL CARE

The International Confederation of Midwives (ICM) essential competencies for pre-conceptual and antenatal midwifery practice (ICM 2018) are presented under the following headings:

1   Provide pre-pregnancy care
2   Determine health status of woman
3   Assess fetal well-being

4   Monitor the progression of pregnancy
5   Promote and support health behaviours that improve well-being
6   Provide anticipatory guidance related to pregnancy, birth and parenthood
7   Detect, stabilise, manage and refer women with complicated pregnancies
8   Assist the woman and her family to plan for an appropriate place of birth
9   Provide care to women with unintended or mistimed pregnancy

These global competencies will be used throughout the chapter to provide a framework to describe the role of the midwife in pre-conceptual and antenatal care.

PRE-CONCEPTUAL CARE

PROVIDE PRE-PREGNANCY CARE

INTRODUCTION

Whilst is would seem sensible and is certainly advisable, the idea of preparing for a pregnancy is by no means a universal consideration. As most pregnancies are unplanned many women begin pregnancy without the benefit of taking steps to increase their chances of a healthy pregnancy and optimum outcome for both themselves and their baby. Even for those pregnancies that are planned, not all women want to disclose that they are thinking of having a baby, for fear of it taking a long time to conceive or 'tempting fate'. Whilst primary care might seem like a more approachable health system, again the time pressures on GP and health centres, with short appointments and a limited availability of health promotion, is equally unappealing. Unfortunately, many women are not aware that there are positive steps they can take to improve their reproductive health and few healthcare practitioners raise the issue opportunistically (Bortolus et al. 2017).

Yet there are many advantages for women if they are able to access and follow pre-conceptual advice before they start trying for a baby. The challenge is getting the evidence out to the women who need it most and then ensuring that there is easy access to the interventions available. Many women turn to the internet, a never sleeping source of information and intrigue, horror stories and personal accounts to uncover the mysteries around pregnancy and birth.

We now know that pre–pregnancy health can also impact on the long-term health of the baby and even generations to come. The following sections reflect the skills and behaviours required to meet the competencies (ICM 2018).

IDENTIFY AND ASSIST IN REDUCING BARRIERS RELATED TO ACCESSING AND USING SEXUAL HEALTH SERVICES

In an ideal world, all women of reproductive age would be able to engage with local services that enable them to access safe and reliable contraception in a non-judgemental environment. They would therefore feel able to discuss pregnancy plans and be advised on how to best prepare for parenthood. In the UK, sexual health services are often provided by practice nurses, who may or may not have been midwives, and who have usually undertaken further qualifications to enable them to undertake the additional skills of cervical cytology, coil fitting and advising on methods of contraception.

ASSESS NUTRITIONAL STATUS, CURRENT IMMUNISATION STATUS AND HEALTH BEHAVIOURS

NUTRITIONAL STATUS

When a woman is planning a pregnancy, this is the ideal time to make changes in advance of conception that will not only enhance her chances of becoming pregnant but also having a healthy baby. One key example is maternal weight. The rise in the prevalence of obesity worldwide is such that it has become a public health concern. In the UK 6 out of 10 women, and 7 out of 10 men, are overweight (NHS Digital 2018). What constitutes a healthy weight is usually categorised by body mass index (BMI), which is calculated when weight in kilograms is divided by the square of a person's height in metres (kg/m2). A healthy weight range is when the BMI is between 18.5 and 24.9, where the risk of disease associated with adiposity is least at a population level (WHO 2019). Being overweight or obese increases the risk of complications throughout the pregnancy continuum, in addition to those a woman may already face irrespective of pregnancy. These risks include: gestational diabetes, obstetric intervention and stillbirth. It is not easy to lose weight to order and success takes having the right mindset and support (Agha et al. 2014).

IMMUNISATIONS

Infants in the UK are offered immunisations throughout childhood that will help prevent potentially debilitating conditions in a developing fetus, including measles, mumps and rubella (MMR). If a woman has missed out on these childhood vaccinations she should be immunised whilst she is using effective contraception. Vaccination should not be undertaken within a month of conception as a precaution, although there are no known risks of receiving the MMR vaccine in pregnancy (PHE 2018).

SUBSTANCE ABUSE

If a woman is a known user of elicit substances the midwife should refer her to a specialist clinic where she can receive expert support and treatment to help her quit her addiction before she becomes pregnant. However, in reality, women who abuse substances may live a chaotic lifestyle that centres around feeding the habit, and this makes them more at risk of unintended pregnancy. Women who use drugs are also more likely to smoke, drink alcohol and have a poor nutritional status, which also puts the fetus at increased risk. Drug use in pregnancy is associated with fetal abnormalities, growth restriction and neonatal and infant behavioural problems (Baston & Durward 2017); therefore, if the woman accesses pre-pregnancy care, the midwife has an important role befriending and supporting her to engage with services that can help her abstain. Drinking alcohol in pregnancy is associated with a condition known as fetal alcohol syndrome (FAS), which can result in learning difficulties, facial abnormalities and low birth weight. It is therefore recommended that women should avoid alcohol if planning a pregnancy as harm could be done before the pregnancy is confirmed (NHS 2017).

EXISTING MEDICAL CONDITION

If a woman has a pre-existing condition, such as epilepsy, she will have been told about the importance of discussing the prospect of pregnancy with her specialist team from adolescence. The need to consider the impact of her regular medication on a developing fetus is paramount yet needs to be carefully balanced between her health and that of her baby. Some drugs, such as valproate for epilepsy, are known to be teratogenic; that is, they can cause serious fetal malformations. However, the consequences of stopping a drug that controls her life-threatening seizures could be equally catastrophic. Therefore, women need to discuss the alternatives with their specialist team so that any change in drug therapy can be closely managed.

Women with diabetes who are thinking of becoming pregnant will similarly need to plan ahead. Tight control of blood sugar levels and optimum BMI can help minimise the risk of congenital abnormalities, premature birth or stillbirth associated with this chronic disease. It is recommended that women have their glycated haemoglobin (HbA1c) checked with the aim of achieving an optimum level before conception and subsequent organogenesis.

Women known to have, or be a carrier for, a hereditary disease are also advised to seek genetic counselling before they become pregnant so that they can consider the options available to them. It may be, for example, that a woman who has a parent with Huntington's disease (HD) can access and consider pre-implantation genetic diagnosis (PIGD). This procedure would involve undergoing in vitro fertilisation (IVF) so that unaffected embryos could be selected and only those be replaced in the womb. Such difficult decisions require time to think through and discuss with family members.

POLLUTION

There are some environmental factors that influence health which women thinking about having a baby can do little about. Air pollution is increasingly being linked to poor health and reduced life expectancy and the effect of exposure during pregnancy through living in close proximity to major roads is growing (Clemente et al. 2019). She can, however, think about changing her route to work or take steps to ensure that her home is smoke-free.

CARRY OUT SCREENING PROCEDURES FOR SEXUALLY TRANSMITTED INFECTIONS AND
CERVICAL CANCER

In the UK, sexual health clinics provide screening for childbearing women who are sexually active. For example, women under 25 years of age can pick up a postal self-screening kit for Chlamydia, test themselves in the privacy of their own home and receive a text message with the result. The programme for cervical cancer does not begin until women are aged 25 years and continues every three years until the age of 64. Women are invited by letter to attend their local general practice or health clinic. However, women who are not already receiving family planning services may be reluctant to attend, so it is important that all those professionals who are in contact with women of childbearing age are mindful of making every contact count (MECC), so that clear messages are conveyed about the importance of timely screening.

PROVIDE COUNSELLING ABOUT NUTRITIONAL SUPPLEMENTS, EXERCISE AND
FAMILY PLANNING

It is recommended that women take a folic acid supplement (400 micrograms) before they become pregnant and until at least 12 weeks gestation. There is overwhelming evidence that this can reduce the risk of the baby developing a neural tube defect (NTD), such as spina bifida, and indeed, in many countries, foods such as bread are routinely fortified with this nutrient. There are also groups of women for whom it is recommended to take a higher dose (5 milligrams) either because of their previous family history or increased risk of congenital abnormalities, including women with a raised BMI, diabetes or epilepsy.

Women should be aware that they *may* be eligible for Healthy Start vitamins, free of charge, if they are pregnant, and these contain folic acid, vitamin C and vitamin D, which is important for bone health. It is recommended that women who are pregnant and who are breastfeeding take 10 micrograms of vitamin D per day, especially if they have dark skin or do not get much exposure to sunlight (NICE 2008). Unless a woman is known to be anaemic, there is little advantage to taking further additional nutritional supplements. Care should be taken to ensure that if a supplement is considered, that it is specific to pregnancy and does not contain vitamin A, which is teratogenic in high doses.

The midwife who works in pre-conceptual care should encourage women to become physically active, if they are not currently, as exercise is associated with greater joint mobility, reduced risk of diabetes and hypertension as well as enhancing a general sense of well-being (PHE 2019). Women who are already active should continue to engage in activity in which there is no danger of 'bumping the bump'.

Midwives need to have a detailed working knowledge of contraceptive choices so that they can provide women with information to make informed decisions about the most appropriate option for them. Whilst the woman is adjusting her lifestyle and preparing for conception she may wish to change to a barrier method of contraception, especially if she has previously been having injections or taking a contraceptive pill. Similarly, if she has a contraceptive implant, this should be removed to give her body time to resume its normal menstrual cycle.

ANTENATAL CARE

DETERMINE HEALTH STATUS OF WOMAN

CONFIRM PREGNANCY AND ESTIMATE GESTATIONAL AGE FROM HISTORY, PHYSICAL EXAM AND ULTRASOUND

EXPECTED DATE OF DELIVERY (EDD)

There are certain key principles that the midwife holds dear. Being able to estimate a woman's expected date of delivery (EDD) or expected date of birth, before a scan can provide a more accurate assessment, is one of the essential elements of a midwife's toolkit.

This date is extremely important for the woman and her family. All her hopes and expectations are framed around anticipating the birth of her baby, when she should tell her family, when to leave work or even when to buy the pram. A full-term pregnancy is defined by health professionals to be 40 weeks (280 days), although it is considered to be within normal parameters between 37 to 42 completed weeks. Only about 4 per cent of babies actually arrive on the EDD.

Screening tests require precise dating as the results are interpreted in relation to gestational age. It is therefore essential that an accurate EDD is determined. It is also important for management of pregnancy; for example, when a pregnancy goes beyond the EDD or when to time an elective caesarean section.

CALCULATING EDD

A midwife can calculate a woman's EDD based on the assumption that a woman has a 28-day menstrual cycle and was having regular periods. Based on the simple formula:

Add 7 days and 9 months to the first day of her last menstrual period (LMP).

So, for example, if her LMP was 21/10/19 her EDD would be 28/7/20.

However, some women have irregular periods, short or long menstrual cycles or simply cannot remember. Calculating the EDD using dates can therefore be imprecise; however, it provides an estimate on which further appointments, such as the first scan visit, can be arranged. Calculating the gestation using the dates method, involves working out the EDD, then using a calendar, working back from that date as '40' until the current date is reached. Alternatively, many midwives carry a gestational wheel, where the dates around the outside can be matched to an arrow pointing at the LMP and another at the EDD; finding the current date will indicate the gestational age of the fetus.

Access to the internet and pregnancy apps makes this counting and wheel using redundant. Simply putting in an LMP, or accessing a woman's electronic records, will generate the EDD and display the gestation. There are a range of apps that a woman can engage with that will send her regular messages about what her developing baby weighs, measures and looks like as the pregnancy progresses.

ESTIMATING GESTATIONAL AGE

There are a range of physical parameters that the midwife uses to estimate gestational age. The uterus is a pelvic organ until 12 weeks gestation when it becomes palpable above the symphysis pubis bone. Further landmarks enable the midwife to estimate approximate gestation; for example, the fundus is palpable midway between the symphysis pubis and the umbilicus at 16 weeks, at the umbilicus at 20–22 weeks and at 32 weeks it is midway between the umbilicus and xiphisternum. There are many factors that the midwife needs to consider when making this estimation, however, including variations due to the possibility of multiple pregnancy, lie of the baby, if the woman has a full bladder and if she is overweight. Additionally, if a woman has felt fetal movements or 'quickening' as this is usually between 16–24 weeks (or earlier in subsequent pregnancies).

CONFIRMING GESTATIONAL AGE

Ultrasonography is now used to confirm a woman's EDD and, when undertaken early in pregnancy, is an accurate and acceptable means of establishing this important baseline. The fetal measurement that is used is from the head to bottom, known as 'crown rump length' (CRL) and in the UK this first ultrasound scan (USS) is performed at about 12 weeks. In the UK, ultrasonography is usually undertaken by radiographers, although increasingly midwives are taking on this additional role as the demand for scans increases and the capacity of the scan departments becomes ever more stretched.

OBTAIN COMPREHENSIVE HEALTH HISTORY

This is the most important meeting and consultation that the midwife has with the woman. It is known as the 'booking history' and involves taking a detailed account of the woman's medical, family, obstetric, current pregnancy and social history. It forms the basis of her future antenatal, labour and postnatal care; it enables the midwife to make the appropriate referrals if she identifies that the woman's pregnancy or birth may not be straightforward. So, for example, if the woman has a history of having had a previous deep vein thrombosis (DVT), this will influence whom the midwife refers her to for care. Pregnancy is a time when there are considerable changes to the circulatory system (see Chapter 1), which makes a woman at increased risk of developing a thrombosis, irrespective of her previous history.

Thrombosis is the leading cause of maternal death in the UK (Knight et al. 2019). Therefore, if a woman already has a susceptibility to adverse clotting events, it is important that she receives prophylactic treatment. If she has a clotting disorder, she will require specialist care and blood monitoring throughout her pregnancy, in accordance with the most recent evidence-based guidance.

In the UK, if a woman has a medical condition, midwives continue to provide care alongside specialist obstetric care. Sometimes, however, the woman can miss out on developing a relationship with her community midwife and benefiting from being introduced to her local community family centre, if she is having mostly hospital antenatal care. Where no known risks are identified at booking, the woman can have midwifery-led care and never need to see a doctor. However, the midwife may need to refer to a doctor during pregnancy if she detects any deviation from good health in either the mother or the baby.

The woman's family history is also important because there may be babies born in the family with hereditary conditions that might increase the chances of her having an affected baby. The midwife will then refer to a specialist for detailed discussion about the diagnostic options available.

Women who have had a previous complicated pregnancy, or poor fetal outcome, may need to have consultant-led care so that a plan can be made to mitigate the risk of future complications. It is important that the woman continues to have midwifery input, however, so that she can be supported to prepare for motherhood, in whatever circumstances this is ultimately achieved.

ASSESS STATUS OF IMMUNISATIONS, AND UPDATE AS INDICATED

Midwives ask women about their immunisation history and if they have not completed the full schedule of childhood immunisations, such as measles, mumps and rubella, are advised to have these after the baby is born. There are some vaccinations that are offered in pregnancy: pertussis (whooping cough) from 16 weeks gestation and seasonal flu vaccination at any gestation. Women can be reluctant to have injections or take medications in pregnancy for fear of the potential impact on their baby. However, the midwife needs to ensure that women understand the importance of these;

having the pertussis injection during pregnancy means that there is time for the antibodies developed to get through to the baby, so that it is born protected from this life-threatening infection. Influenza is also a serious illness, but in pregnancy women are at increased risk of developing pneumonia if they contract it. Any febrile illness also increases her risk of miscarriage.

OBTAIN BIOLOGICAL SAMPLES FOR LABORATORY TESTS

The midwife is trained to take a range of samples to screen for current or developing pathology. Urinalysis for protein is part of each antenatal assessment, as it may be suggestive of developing pre-eclampsia or urinary tract infection (UTI). Blood is taken to check for blood group and rhesus factor. It is important that the midwife knows a woman's rhesus status, because if the woman is rhesus negative and her baby is rhesus positive, there is a potential risk that any feto-maternal transfusion could lead the woman to make antibodies (sensitisation) (NICE 2016). This risk increases following trauma to the abdomen or during an invasive procedure such as amniocentesis. Whilst not so dangerous for the first pregnancy, if she started a subsequent pregnancy already with antibodies that could attack the developing fetal blood cells, the pregnancy would be at serious risk of developing a condition called haemolytic disease of the fetus and newborn (HDFN). For this reason, in the UK, rhesus negative women with a known rhesus positive fetus are offered a prophylactic anti-D injection at around 28–30 weeks to prevent the development of antibodies (NICE 2008). Also, if women do have a sensitising event, they are advised to seek care so that blood can be taken to establish if fetal cells have entered her blood stream and additional anti-D offered.

Blood is also taken to establish the woman's iron status and if she needs treatment to prevent her becoming iron depleted. Anaemia in pregnancy is not only associated with the unpleasant symptoms of breathlessness and fatigue, but is also linked with complications such as post-partum haemorrhage. It is important therefore that the midwife helps prevent this potential life-threatening condition, by screening during pregnancy, supporting the woman to take any iron supplements prescribed and informs her which foods are rich in iron.

Women who live in countries where conditions such as sickle cell disease and thalassaemia are prevalent are offered screening by 10 weeks. If the woman is identified as a carrier, it is advisable that the father of the baby is also counselled and offered screening to determine the risk to the fetus; this situation needs a sensitive approach by the midwife because if he is also a carrier there is a one-in-four chance that the baby may inherit the disease.

In the UK, all women are offered screening for syphilis, hepatitis and HIV during pregnancy so that if infection is detected, treatment can be offered, thus reducing the risk of transmission to the fetus.

PROVIDE INFORMATION ABOUT CONDITIONS THAT MAY BE DETECTED BY SCREENING

Antenatal screening for fetal conditions is offered in the first trimester, through a combination of blood and ultrasound investigations. The conditions routinely screened for include Down's syndrome, Edwards' syndrome and Patau's syndrome. It is essential that the woman and her partner are aware of the options available; the midwife has an important role in explaining what the blood tests are for, how she will get the results, what the results mean and what options are then available. They should be aware that screening tests are to find out if the mother has a higher chance of having a health problem; they do not diagnose it. Not all women will want to go down the route of screening, whereas others may want to have the initial screening and then take it from there. In the UK, results are presented as a 'higher chance' or 'lower chance' with a threshold of over 1 in 150 considered low chance. So, for example, if the Down's risk may come back as 1:149, the woman would be counselled about the diagnostic options. This issue needs careful consideration as there is also a potential risk of miscarriage with amniocentesis or chorionic villus sampling of approximately 0.5–1 per cent, so these risks need to be carefully weighed against whether or not having a child with a genetic condition is something that the couple could contemplate.

SCREENING FOR MENTAL ILLNESS AND EMOTIONAL DISTRESS

Women are also screened regarding their mental health status. In the UK, women are asked a range of questions designed to identify symptoms of depression and also anxiety (NICE 2008). If this screening is positive, women may be referred back to their family doctor or to a range of self-help tools such as IAPT. Women with a history of severe mental illness, such as psychosis or bipolar disorder, or women with current mental health concerns, will be referred to a perinatal mental health service for expert assessment, care planning and follow up.

Women may come to pregnancy having had a range of Adverse Childhood Experiences (ACEs); a phrase adopted by Felitti et al. (1998) to describe a range of events which can have an enduring impact on the way people see the world and process their experiences. These ACEs include emotional, physical and sexual abuse and being raised in a home where they witness domestic violence, substance abuse or parental separation. ACEs not only impact on emotional health but can lead to deterioration in physical health and an increased risk of substance abuse, violent crime and incarceration (Bellis et al. 2015). The impact of ACEs, however, can be mitigated by the presence of an emotionally available adult, and there are techniques, such as Video Interaction Guidance (VIG), that can be used by specialist health visitors and child and adolescent mental health workers with parents to help them connect and develop close relationships with their baby or child.

Midwives have a valuable role to play in breaking the cycle, so that babies of mothers who have experienced adversity do not then fall victim to neglect or emotional and physical trauma. Asking 'What has happened to you?' rather than 'What is wrong with you?' can elicit information that can help midwives understand the mother's perspective and where she can be referred to for help. Trauma-informed care is a model that is now forming and developing in the UK for practitioners across many social and healthcare sectors and NHS Education Scotland is leading the way providing valuable models and educational resources.

DISCUSS FINDINGS AND POTENTIAL IMPLICATIONS WITH WOMAN AND MUTUALLY DETERMINE PLAN OF CARE

The midwife not only counsels for screening tests, but needs to have a detailed knowledge of the implications of positive results and the subsequent action that might be offered to the woman. Together they can work out a plan of care that is acceptable to all. Not all women respond to treatments in the same way; for example, some women will cope well with oral iron therapy and others may not. Therefore, the midwife needs to regularly review any programmes of treatment with the woman, to check they are tolerable and being followed. Repeat testing and monitoring of the success of the treatment will also be required and the midwife is responsible for ensuring this happens and referring for medical input if the condition does not respond.

PERFORM A COMPLETE PHYSICAL EXAMINATION

Attending hospital for antenatal care may be the first time that a woman has ever set foot inside a hospital facility. Likewise, she may not have accessed health services since she was vaccinated as a child. Pregnancy presents an opportunity for some women across the world to have their heart and lungs auscultated (listened to), have a cervical smear or have blood pressure (BP) and urine checked. In the UK, routine newborn and infant screening and comprehensive national healthcare means that many of the women that attend for pregnancy care will have had major physical conditions ruled out, therefore a clinical examination of heart and lungs is no longer part of routine antenatal care.

Many women will have had their blood pressure taken as part of contraception care; however, this important screening test takes on a new dimension in pregnancy as it will be taken now at every antenatal visit as part of screening for pre-eclampsia. This is a condition that affects about 6 per cent of pregnancies and is more common in women who have a family history of it. It is characterised by raised blood pressure, proteinuria and the sudden development of oedema (swelling) and if untreated can result in the woman developing eclampsia, where the woman has life-threatening convulsions and an abnormal blood profile. NICE guidance (NICE 2008) recommends that all pregnant women should be informed of the danger signs of developing pre-eclampsia.

ASSESS FETAL WELL-BEING

ASSESS FETAL WELL-BEING THROUGH EXAMINATION OF THE MATERNAL ABDOMEN

Although the advent of ultrasound has given us a window onto the world of the developing fetus, most women will only have two scans during their pregnancy, at 12 and 20 weeks gestation. Those at high risk of fetal growth compromise (for example, previous small baby or diabetes), or where it is difficult to monitor the fetus in other ways, for example when a woman has excess adipose tissue, will have additional scans as part of their pathway of care.

ASSESS FETAL SIZE

The midwife uses her clinical dexterity to estimate fetal size and growth. When she palpates the woman's abdomen, the midwife uses a range of landmarks combined with measuring the distance between the symphysis pubis (bone at the front of the pelvis) and the fundus (top of the uterus) to establish appropriate growth for gestational age. The midwife will refer the woman for a growth scan if she detects reduced growth. Occasionally the midwife may detect increased amniotic fluid during abdominal palpation, or have difficulty assessing growth if the woman has excess adipose tissue, and again she will need to refer her for an ultrasonography assessment.

ASSESS PRESENTATION

In the third trimester of pregnancy, it is important that the midwife can identify the presentation (head or bottom first) of the fetus, on abdominal palpation, so that care can be planned accordingly. The midwife learns this skill under supervision during her pre-registration training. She also learns how to assess if the presenting part is descending into the pelvis, which way the baby is facing and how to listen to the fetal heart. Locating and listening to the fetal heart can provide the midwife with corroborating information about the baby's position as it is heard loudest over the back of the fetal shoulder.

ASSESS FETAL MOVEMENTS AND ASK WOMAN ABOUT FETAL ACTIVITY

Monitoring fetal well-being includes encouraging the woman to tune into the baby's movements and become aware of its activity and rest times, identify kicks, stretches, hiccups and rolls. Women should know when and how to report episodes of reduced fetal movements. It is important that the midwife responds positively to such incidents, so that the woman does not become discouraged or feel stupid to do this on more than one occasion and delay making contact again. Reduced fetal movements are associated with fetal compromise and repeated episodes may require intervention to deliver the baby sooner rather than later.

MONITOR THE PROGRESSION OF PREGNANCY

CONDUCT ASSESSMENTS OF WOMAN'S PHYSICAL AND PSYCHOLOGICAL WELL-BEING

The World Health Organization (WHO 2016) recommends that all women access antenatal care at least four times during their pregnancy, although globally compliance was only 64 per cent up to 2014. This number of attendances is an absolute minimum and most women value additional contact with their midwife. In the UK, the schedule of care is determined by NICE Guidance (NICE 2008), which stipulates ten visits for first-time mothers and seven for multiparous women. Each visit has a particular remit, but all include blood pressure and urine testing and asking the woman how she is feeling both physically and emotionally. Whilst the initial phases of antenatal care are about risk assessment and screening for potential abnormality, the latter is more about preparation for parenthood and detecting any developing pathology.

Whilst the physical checks are important, considering a woman's emotional well-being must have equal credence. In the PINK study (Baston 2006), one woman, 'Elizabeth', recalled that she had been apprehensive about the birth throughout her pregnancy because of her previous birth experience:

> I just felt like something was going to go wrong … I don't know, because like he'd gone over, and I didn't even have any twinges or anything to – I just wanted it all done [...] I was just like a big beached whale sat on the settee not able to move. And, and that fortnight of just sitting and thinking, you know, 'What's going to happen? What's going to happen?' Stupid really, I should have just got on with it and not sort of thought about it (87).

But when she raised her fears with the midwife, whilst she was listened to, her concerns were not truly heard. She felt frustrated because no one took her fears seriously.

It is common for midwives to 'reassure' women but this often happens in a way that does not acknowledge that the woman is voicing a genuine concern which needs to be heard. In the example above, the midwife was theoretically correct, that second labours and births are usually quicker. However, that cannot be guaranteed. The midwives caring for 'Elizabeth' could have asked what was it about her previous experience that had been so difficult, listen to her story and then offer to plan for ways to help address those specific concerns. This would have helped Elizabeth feel that she had someone alongside her, who understood how she felt and genuinely wanted to help make the situation better. This is how midwives can provide compassionate care.

Other situations that can impact on a woman's emotional wellbeing are her social networks and those she can seek support from. Relationships with family members can change during pregnancy and the midwife as advocate and befriender has a role in protecting women from avoidable harm. Women should be given the opportunity during pregnancy to disclose domestic violence (DV). It may take several times before a woman will disclose that she has a violent partner and therefore she should be asked on a number of occasions. The midwife also needs to vigilant to the signs of DV, as many women do not reveal their situations for fear of reprisal or social service involvement.

PROVIDE INFORMATION REGARDING NORMAL PREGNANCY PROGRESS

Women should know what to expect during pregnancy so that they do not make assumptions about what is normal. For example, for years old wives' tales have perpetuated myths such as, the baby starts to slow down with its movements towards the end of pregnancy. Such myths need dispelling so that the woman can make wise choices and decisions according to her unique circumstances. The midwife should make sure that the woman knows that she can continue to exercise safely, does not need to eat for two, and what to expect when labour starts.

PROVIDE INFORMATION (INCLUDING WRITTEN AND/OR PICTORIAL) ABOUT DANGER SIGNS

It is also part of the midwives' role to make sure that the woman knows when she should contact her midwife; for example, if she experiences any bleeding, if her waters break or if she has any headaches or visual disturbances. If she experiences any contractions before 37 weeks of pregnancy or abdominal pain that is constant, she should contact the maternity unit immediately. Early intervention can help prevent a tragedy occurring and the woman should feel sufficiently confident to approach her midwife if she has any concerns or questions during her pregnancy.

SUGGEST MEASURES TO COPE WITH COMMON DISCOMFORTS OF PREGNANCY

Woman can experience a range of normal but potentially unpleasant disorders during pregnancy. Information, support and a kind listening ear may go a long way to helping her cope with these. For example, it is not unusual for women to experience indigestion especially in the last trimester as the growing uterus occupies the space where the stomach used to sit unimpeded. The midwife can provide simple remedies, such as avoiding spicy foods, sitting upright and having an extra pillow in bed to help prevent gastric reflux. Simple antacids can also be useful to help neutralise the burning sensations when the acidic contents of the stomach leak back into the oesophagus.

The midwife must also use her knowledge to differentiate between symptoms that might reflect a common disorder versus something more serious. For example, if a woman is experiencing breathlessness on exertion, the midwife must ensure that the woman is not anaemic or that its onset was not sudden or severe, suggestive of possible pulmonary hypertension or associated with pain suggestive of a pulmonary embolism. Only then can it be attributed to the growing uterus taking up some of the space the diaphragm uses to facilitate deep breathing, and even so, the midwife should review how the woman is feeling at subsequent visits, to feel confident that all is still well. The woman can be reassured that, usually, as the fetal head starts to descend into the pelvis in those last weeks of pregnancy, a little more space under the woman's ribs literally gives her some light relief to breathe more easily, a phenomenon known as 'lightening'.

There are many other minor disorders of pregnancy that the midwife can help the woman to resolve for herself. They include: giving information about how to prevent and treat constipation through dietary advice; assisting with the relief of varicose veins through suggestions about exercise, leg elevation and use of support tights; offering information about getting comfortable in bed to aid restful sleep; and many more. Whilst offering advice is helpful, the empathy and active listening involved in hearing about women's problems is in itself therapeutic.

REVIEW FINDINGS AND REVISE PLAN OF CARE WITH WOMAN AS PREGNANCY PROGRESSES

As the pregnancy progresses the woman and the midwife may need to change the original plans to accommodate a change in need. The midwife may detect, during an antenatal check-up, that the fetus is no longer presenting head first but is presenting by the breech. The midwife would then need to explain the options available to the woman so that a new plan can be put in place. For example, women who have straightforward pregnancies but a breech presentation should be offered the option of having the baby turned, a procedure known as 'External Cephalic Version' (ECV). Performed at the maternity unit by a skilled practitioner, this should only be performed under scan guidance to prevent cord entanglement and to confirm that a cephalic presentation is not inadvertently turned to become a breech. There is also a small chance of bleeding or fetal distress so this should only be performed when the pregnancy is at full term and with the option of having an emergency caesarean section urgently should any complication arise. The woman would also need to know what would happen if ECV was not successful and in what circumstances a vaginal breech birth might be possible. Changes to the plan of care might need to be accommodated such as changing from a home birth to a planned caesarean section if a vaginal breech is contraindicated for some reason.

PROMOTE AND SUPPORT HEALTH BEHAVIOURS THAT IMPROVE WELL-BEING

PROVIDE EMOTIONAL SUPPORT TO WOMEN TO ENCOURAGE CHANGE IN HEALTH BEHAVIOUR

The midwife has an important role in public health as pregnancy is a window of opportunity to support women to adopt a lifestyle that will give her and her family optimum health. Whenever the midwife is contemplating providing the woman with guidance in any area related to her health and well-being, she needs to consider the most appropriate approach. One option to consider is motivational interviewing, which is a counselling approach designed by psychologists Miller and Rollnick (1991). It uses a client-centred approach to facilitate behaviour change through its central purpose of resolving ambivalence, by eliciting 'change talk' via the use of open-ended questions, reflective listening and summarising. There are five key principles to MI: expressing empathy so the woman feels heard and respected; developing discrepancy between the woman's current self and future self; avoiding arguments so the woman does not become defensive; meeting resistance with professionalism; and enhancing self-efficacy by building on the woman's strengths, which can be used in future plans for behaviour change.

PROVIDE INFORMATION TO WOMAN AND FAMILY ABOUT IMPACT ON MOTHER AND FETUS OF RISK CONDITIONS

Some areas of behaviour change require specialist support and additional time, therefore it may be that the role of the woman's named midwife is to raise the issue and signpost to care. The term 'Very Brief Advice' (VBA) has been used to describe a quick intervention that can be used in any consultation by any member of staff, to ensure patients are referred for dedicated support. VBA comprises: Ask, Advise and Act and, in relation to smoking in pregnancy, relates to asking the woman about her smoking status, advising her she is four times more likely to successfully quit smoking with trained support and asking her if she would like to be referred to a smoking cessation specialist. NICE (2010) guidelines, however, recommend that midwives offer carbon monoxide (CO) screening to all women at booking and all subsequent appointments. Being able to respond to a raised CO reading provides information to the woman about how her own smoking is impacting on her health. Not all readings are raised because the woman smokes; it may be that she is exposed to passive smoke by a member of the household, or that there is a faulty gas appliance that is responsible for the CO in her system. Smoking cessation services will be further explored in Chapter 8.

COUNSEL WOMEN ABOUT AND OFFER REFERRAL FOR ASSISTANCE AND TREATMENT

Whilst the midwife is the lead professional for women experiencing a straightforward pregnancy, there will be times when she needs to refer women to another professional or more senior colleague for advice or treatment. Examples include: perinatal mental health team, if the woman has a history of severe mental illness; diabetes team, if the woman had previous gestational or existing diabetes; or a physiotherapist, if a woman is experiencing symphysis pubis dysfunction. The woman will still continue to receive care form her community midwife, whilst liaising and consulting with additional specialisms. Some women experience a severe fear of childbirth or tokophobia (Aksoy et al. 2015) and will benefit from referral to a senior midwife or psychologist who can help them resolve their fear or find a solution that enables them to continue their pregnancy with the knowledge that there is a personal plan of care in place.

RESPECT WOMEN'S DECISIONS ABOUT PARTICIPATING IN TREATMENTS AND PROGRAMMES

We are all unique and no more so than when making decisions about maternity care. The midwife will therefore have her own personal views about what she might accept if she were pregnant and the choices she would make, but she cannot expect each woman to make similar choices. The midwife must feel assured that the woman understands the implications for her choices but cannot make them for her. If the woman declines antenatal screening for Down's syndrome, for example, that is her choice. She may also have particular religious views, such as a Jehovah's Witness not accepting a blood transfusion, which the midwife will need to carefully discuss and document with the woman and make contingencies for, but never judge.

PROVIDE ANTICIPATORY GUIDANCE RELATED TO PREGNANCY, BIRTH AND PARENTHOOD

PARTICIPATE IN AND REFER WOMEN AND SUPPORT PERSONS TO CHILDBIRTH EDUCATION PROGRAMMES

There are a range of childbirth and parent education opportunities available to women, depending on their needs, where they live and what they can afford. Some women access education sessions provided by the local maternity unit, facilitated by midwives, to gain insight into what is available. Usually, these sessions are only offered to women and their partners during the first pregnancy because of limited availability. Traditionally, such courses ran over a series of weeks, enabling the participants to develop friendships and support networks. However, due to financial pressures on statutory health services, many of these have now been squeezed into concentrated day or weekend programmes and are often oversubscribed. For women who can pay, there are private classes which provide the benefits of small group sessions over a series of weeks, fulfilling the remits of valuable social support for new parents, often for many years to come. Women who have been identified with particular parenting needs may be referred to specific programmes (see 'Parenting programmes' under Resources) to assist them to develop skills and strategies to cope with the challenges of caring for their infant.

PLANNING FOR THE BIRTH

Throughout antenatal care the midwife will be incorporating information and advice about the impending birth and care of the baby. Planning for birth usually takes a more formal course in the last trimester of pregnancy when the midwife will aim to try and see the woman in her own home and discuss her hopes and fears for the labour and strategies to help her achieve or overcome them. Formal birth planning, where the discussion is documented, provides an opportunity for aspects of care to be considered at a time when the woman is not in labour, when it would be more difficult to consider and weigh up what she feels is right for her. So, for example, the midwife will ask the woman what she would prefer to happen during the third stage of labour; either to wait and let nature take its course to expel the placenta, or to have an injection of oxytocin which will reduce the length of the third stage and potentially the amount of blood lost. Raising the issue therefore gives the woman time to think about what she wants to do, to ask further questions of the midwife and to discuss it with her partner if she wishes.

Other issues raised during the birth planning visit include: how the woman wants to cope with the contractions; what positions she wants to be in to give birth; who she wants to have with her as birth companions; and information about the vitamin K injection for the baby.

Coping with contractions in labour is an issue that needs careful consideration by the woman, and the midwife can help her explore the options and the reality. In the PINK study (Baston 2006) one woman, 'Sara', described how she wished she had known how painful it was going to be so that she could have prepared herself for it:

> I don't know whether you can prepare for it or not, but I had no understanding just how difficult it was going to be. So, erm, and I felt absolutely exhausted afterwards. And in a way slightly let down because I'd built myself up to the fact that I was going to have this baby naturally, and I was going to go for limited pain relief – when in the end I ended up with erm, an emergency section (81).

The reality of childbirth and parenthood can come as a huge upheaval to women who are not prepared. Talking through what to expect on a one-to-one basis is the ideal scenario, as the specific impact on a particular woman will be unique to her. Information can be tailored by the midwife for her specific circumstances. In the PINK study (Baston 2006) one woman, 'Rachel', described how she found that she was emotionally labile in the weeks following the birth. She put this down to the fact that she had an exciting and demanding career before her daughter was born:

> I'm used to being a, a manager at work. I'm used to having a job which is intellectually stimulating [...] I'm used to asking someone to do something for me and it gets done. And all of a sudden, you've got this thing that won't do as you want it to (laughter) who gets you up three times a night for a feed [...] it's just such a shock (77).

THINKING ABOUT FEEDING

For many women, the birth will be the most overwhelming feature of their preparative thinking. Yet midwives have a crucial role in preparing women for feeding their baby and helping them develop close and loving relationships with their baby while they are pregnant. The Baby Friendly Initiative (BFI) (UNICEF 2019) recommends a 'guiding approach' (4) in order to keep conversations woman centred. The emphasis has moved away from providing the woman with a long list of the benefits of breastfeeding, to finding out what she already knows, what her experiences of infant feeding have been and showing empathy to her situation. When it is appropriate the midwife can then ask permission to give her information to help fill in any gaps or misconceptions. Whichever feeding method the woman is considering, all women should be encouraged to notice their unborn baby's movement patterns, to stroke their tummy and talk to their baby. There should be open conversations about skin-to-skin contact at birth and responsive feeding.

PREPARE THE WOMAN, PARTNER AND FAMILY TO RECOGNISE LABOUR ONSET AND WHEN TO SEEK CARE

A woman must know when and how to contact the maternity unit when she thinks she might be in labour. Considerations such as regular uterine contractions that are getting closer together and lasting longer and feeling that she needs some support are all important. However, whilst the midwife can give a range of parameters for the woman to consider, judging when a woman is in established labour uses all of the midwife's senses. It is therefore important that the woman rings the maternity unit for advice. She will get through to a midwife who will ask her a range of questions so that she can assess if the woman needs to come in straightaway or if she can stay at home for now and enjoy the benefits of her own creature comforts for longer. During the time that the midwife is speaking to her – asking her when her baby is due, if everything has been straightforward so far, has she had any bleeding or loss of fluid and is the baby active – she will also be assessing the tone of the woman's voice and how many times she has had to stop speaking due to a contraction. It is this combined assessment of maternal and fetal well-being that will enable the midwife to suggest the best course of action for that woman.

Women should know that they should always seek immediate care if they have any bleeding, contractions before they are 37 weeks, loss of fluid, pain that is constant, reduced fetal movements, visual disturbances or if they just do not feel right.

There ae many situations in the antenatal period where the midwife needs to be sure she has provided timely and appropriate information to women to support their decision-making. These include issues already raised such as antenatal screening, what not to eat, what supplements to take and choosing place of birth. Sometimes the topic is clear cut, such as, contact the midwife if you think your waters have gone, and others are more complex and need tailoring to individual circumstances.

An example of providing simple information in complex circumstances might arise when the midwife discusses with the parents where the baby is going to sleep. It is important that they understand the basic principles of safer sleeping antenatally, so that they can prepare their home accordingly. For example, parents need to be aware that the safest place for the baby to sleep in the first six months of the baby's life is in a cot in the same room as its parents. The house should be smoke-free and the room should be between 16 and 20 degrees centigrade. The mattress should be firm and the surface washable; there should be no cot bumpers and light blankets should be used rather than a duvet. Raising these issues can be complex especially with women in cultures where it is traditional for the baby to be heavily swaddled and the parents usually share a bed with other children. The house may be overbearingly warm and smoky. The midwife must therefore be diplomatic in the way that she explains that the baby should not be overwrapped and its head should be uncovered as not overheating the baby has been shown to reduce the risk of stillbirth.

DETECT, STABILISE, MANAGE AND REFER WOMEN WITH COMPLICATED PREGNANCIES

The midwife may be the first health professional to identify a complication or cause for concern. She therefore needs to be able to take swift and appropriate action to facilitate the implementation of expert care. As the midwife works in a variety of settings she will need to make best use of the resources that she has. So, for example, if she detects a cord prolapse while undertaking a stretch and sweep procedure at a children's centre, she will need to summon emergency paramedic support for immediate transfer into the maternity unit, whilst endeavouring to keep the presenting part from crushing the cord and cutting off the baby's blood supply. However, if the midwife was in the maternity unit at the time, she would be able to summon additional support, including the option of saline infusion to fill the bladder to support the presenting part and recourse to emergency caesarean section if the cervix was not fully dilated.

Other antenatal emergencies that might potentially arise during antenatal care include: pre-eclampsia, antepartum haemorrhage, fetal distress, psychosis and severe anxiety. There may also be other urgent situations that require immediate referral to obstetric care, whilst the midwife stabilises and monitors the woman's condition.

ASSIST THE WOMAN AND HER FAMILY TO PLAN FOR AN APPROPRIATE PLACE OF BIRTH

DISCUSS OPTIONS, PREFERENCES AND CONTINGENCY PLANS WITH WOMAN AND RESPECT THEIR DECISION

Making plans for the place of birth often begins before conception; the woman may choose where she has her baby based on recommendations from family or friends and also depending on the nearest available facility. The midwife has a key role in presenting the options in such a way that the woman feels she can make her own choice. This is dependent, however, on the midwife feeling confident with all the options. For example, the midwife needs to feel confident to support a home birth, to have observed and facilitated it to really appreciate what a fulfilling experience it can be for both the family and the midwife.

The midwife needs to be able to present the options in a balanced way. Often maternity services will have a website or information leaflet about how the various options differ and the advantages and disadvantages of each. For example, if a woman has her heart set on an epidural for pain relief in labour, then a consultant-led option would be the most appropriate or only choice. However, if she wanted a pool birth, there may be the option to rent a pool for a home birth or use the facilities at the nearest birth centre. Other factors also play a part; for example, if the woman had a previous quick labour, she might want to ask her community midwife to assess her labour progress at home when she has the first signs of labour. Alternatively, a woman may have had a previous traumatic experience in the maternity unit and choose to go elsewhere or stay at home.

If the woman has had a previous birth complication or has a high-risk pregnancy, such as expecting twins or has a breech presentation, the midwife will explain why it might be appropriate to plan for a birth in a maternity unit where there can be swift recourse to emergency caesarean if a serious situation develops.

When choosing place of birth, the available evidence should be considered. There are a range of options available: consultant-led unit (CLU); midwifery-led unit (MLU) (either free-standing or alongside a CLU); or home birth. The evidence (Kurinczuk et al. 2015) suggests that:

- woman having their first baby and planning a home birth or in an MLU have an increased risk of adverse outcome for their baby, although they will experience fewer interventions;
- women having their second or subsequent baby at home or in an MLU have fewer interventions with no increased risk to their baby.

However, the risks are individual to the woman, where she lives, her age, ethnicity, what the local resources are and transfer time to the CLU. Sometimes the midwife and woman might discuss the options but not decide on a fixed option until later in the pregnancy, perhaps even electing to decide when she goes into labour. Women who plan to have a home birth should know what options will be available for pain relief, how long it might take for an ambulance transfer and when she might be asked to change her plans and go into the maternity unit. Transfer in may be advised in situations where there is fetal distress, raised blood pressure or elevated maternal temperature, the need for additional pain relief or simply delay at any stage.

It is important that the woman's partner is also included in discussions as they may feel particularly vulnerable when contemplating a home birth. It is essential that the woman is able to relax during labour without also worrying about how her partner is coping, so there needs to be open and frank discussion and listening to each other's point of view to find an agreeable solution.

Consideration should also be given regarding distance from the maternity unit, how the woman will get there and how long it might take. When women live remotely, such as rural or island locations, there needs to be considerable planning for a few weeks ahead of the birth. In some of the Hebridean islands, for example, it is usual practice for the woman to plan to stay on the mainland, from about 37 weeks. This can be particularly difficult if the woman has other children and has to contemplate leaving them behind. Also, separation from family and friends at such an important time in her life can be isolating and difficult to bear. There will be women who therefore choose not to leave home and will rely on the skills and care of the local community midwifery service and the air-sea rescue service if transfer to the mainland is required. Therefore, preparing women to have optimum health in readiness for the rigours of birth is paramount.

PROVIDE CARE TO WOMEN WITH UNINTENDED OR MISTIMED PREGNANCY

During the course of providing midwifery care, midwives will inevitably encounter situations where the woman is not overjoyed to be pregnant, or sadly may be devastated to have the news confirmed. The midwife must remain non-judgemental, impartial and provide women with the information about what options are available, and where and how to access them. In the UK, there are specialist gynaecological services to provide termination of pregnancy (TOP) counselling in more depth. It is therefore usual for the midwife to refer the woman for counselling, to discuss the medical versus surgical options available for termination of the pregnancy and to meet the necessary legal requirements for this to take place. If the woman decides to continue with the pregnancy, she will need compassionate care to help her bond with her baby in utero or to contemplate adoption, referring to the appropriate social services for ongoing support.

In some health systems, the midwife is a member of the team providing counselling for termination of pregnancy. It is paramount that the woman stays safe and is not inclined to access illegal abortion services in order to achieve the outcome that she feels is best for her. NICE (2019) recommend that women should be able to self-refer to abortion services and that information should be readily available for women to access.

CONCLUSION

The midwife must master a range of complex clinical and social interactional skills to provide bespoke woman-centred care in pregnancy. The evidence base supporting antenatal care provision is constantly changing and maternity services need to keep pace in order to ensure that safe and effective care is on offer. The midwife has a fundamental role in ensuring that women have a positive pregnancy experience through the way that she communicates, interacts, listens to and hears what women hope from their pregnancies.

RESOURCES

Cervical screening. What is cervical screening? www.nhs.uk/con ditions/cervical-screening/. This resource uses simple language and an animated video to talk through the procedure for having screening and getting results.

Diabetes UK. Planning for a pregnancy when you have diabetes, www.diabetes.org.uk/guide-to-diabetes/life-with-diabetes/pregna ncy. Useful information presented in videos, patient stories and clinical information for women with diabetes.

Epilepsy action. Planning a baby, www.epilepsy.org.uk/info/da ily-life/having-baby/planning. This website provides detailed information about the risks and benefits of various medications and the importance of pre-pregnancy counselling.

Healthy Start, www.healthystart.nhs.uk. Website with information about what vitamins to take in pregnancy and breastfeeding, how to apply for them and to check for local retailers.

Huntington's Disease Association, www.hda.org.uk/hunting tons-disease. Website with resources for patients and professionals and latest research summaries.

Motivational Interviewing, https://motivationalinterviewing. org/motivational-interviewing-resources. This extensive resource, hosted by the Motivational Interviewing Network of Trainers

(MINT), includes a library of research papers, videos, assessment tools and presentations.

Parenting programmes, www.fph.org.uk/policy-campaigns/sp ecial-interest-groups/special-interest-groups-list/public-mental-hea lth-special-interest-group/better-mental-health-for-all/a-good-sta rt-in-life/parenting-programmes/. Faculty of public health. This website includes detailed information about a range of programmes including: Watch, Wait and Wonder; Family Nurse Partnership; Incredible Years; Triple P; Mellow Parenting; etc.

Preconception. What is preconception care? www.nhs.uk/ common-health-questions/pregnancy/what-is-preconception-ca re/. NHS resource with additional links to specific subjects such as: screening; questions about pregnancy; increasing chances of pregnancy; fertility; etc.

Trauma-informed care. NHS Education for Scotland (NES) (2017). Transforming Psychological Trauma: A Knowledge and Skills Framework for the Scottish Workforce, www.nes.scot.nhs. uk/media/3971582/nationaltraumatrainingframework.pdf.

Video Interaction Guidance (VIG) Association for Video Interaction Guidance UK, www.videointeractionguidance.net/about vig. A range of research resources and videos explaining the technique.

REFERENCES

Agha M, Agha R, and Sandal J (2014). Interventions to reduce and prevent obesity in pre-conceptual and pregnant women: a systematic review and meta-analysis. *PLoS ONE* 9(5):E95132.

Aksoy A, Ozkan H, and Gundogdu G (2015). Fear of childbirth in women with normal pregnancy evolution. *Clin Exp Obstet Gynecol.* 42:179–183.

Baston H (2006). Women's experience of emergency caesarean birth. PhD thesis. University of York, http://etheses.whiterose.ac.uk/14082/.

Baston H, and Durward H (2017). *Examination of the newborn: a practical guide.* 3rd ed. Oxon: Routledge.

Bellis M, Ashton K, Hughes K, *et al.* (2015). Adverse childhood experiences and their impact on health harming behaviours in the Welsh adult population, www2.nphs.wales.nhs.uk:8080/PRIDDocs.nsf/7c21215d6d0c613e80256f49 0030c05a/d488a3852491bc1d80257f370038919e/$FILE/ACE%20Report% 20FINAL%20(E).pdf. Accessed 26 October 2019.

Bortolus R, Oprandi NC, Rech Morassutti F, *et al.* (2017). Why women do not ask for information on preconception health? A qualitative study. *BMC Pregnancy Childbirth* 17(1):5.

Clemente D, Vrijheid M, Martens D, *et al.* (2019). Prenatal and childhood traffic-related air pollution exposure and telomere length in European children: the HELIX project. *Environmental Health Perspectives* 127(8), doi:10.1289/EHP4148.

Felitti V, Anda R, Nordenberg D, *et al.* (1998). Relationship of childhood abuse and household dysfunction to many of the leading causes of death in adults. The adverse childhood experiences (ACE) study. *American Journal of Preventative Medicine* 14(4):245–258.

Heazall A, Budd J, Thompson J, *et al.* (2017). Association between maternal sleep practices and late stillbirth – findings from a stillbirth case-control study. *BJOG* 125(2):254–262.

ICM (International Confederation of Midwives) (2018). Essential competencies for midwifery practice, www.internationalmidwives.org/assets/files/general-files/2019/03/icm-competencies-en-screens.pdf.

Knight M, Bunch K, Tuffnell D, *et al.* (Eds) on behalf of MBRRACE-UK (2019). *Saving lives, improving mothers' care – lessons learned to inform maternity care from the UK and Ireland confidential enquiries into maternal deaths and morbidity 2014–2016.* Oxford: National Perinatal Epidemiology Unit, University of Oxford.

Kurinczuk J, Knight M, and Hollowell J (Eds) (2015). Evidence review to support the National Maternity Review 2015. Report 1: summary of the evidence on safety of place of birth; and implications for policy and practice from the overall evidence review. Oxford: National Perinatal Epidemiology Unit, University of Oxford. www.england.nhs.uk/wp-content/uploads/2015/07/npeu-report1-safety-of-birthplace-and-implications.pdf.

Miller W, and Rollnick S (1991). *Motivational interviewing: preparing people to change addictive behavior.* New York: Guilford Press.

NHS (2017). Fetal alcohol syndrome, www.nhs.uk/conditions/foetal-alcohol-syndrome/. Accessed 23 October 2019.

NHS Digital (2018). Health Survey for England 2017, https://digital.nhs.uk/data-and-information/publications/statistical/health-survey-for-england. Accessed 11 August 2019.

NICE (National Institute for Health and Care Excellence) (2008, updated 2019). Antenatal care: for uncomplicated pregnancies. CG62, www.nice.org.uk/guidance/cg62/chapter/1-Guidance. Accessed 23 October 2019.

NICE (National Institute for Health and Care Excellence) (2010). Smoking: stopping in pregnancy and after childbirth. Public health guideline [PH26], www.nice.org.uk/guidance/ph26. Accessed 27 October 2019.

NICE (National Institute for Health and Care Excellence) (2016). High-throughput non-invasive prenatal testing for fetal RHD genotype. Diagnostics guidance [DG25], www.nice.org.uk/guidance/dg25/chapter/1-Recomm endations. Accessed 24 October 2019.

NICE (National Institute for Health and Care Excellence) (2019). Abortion care NG140, www.nice.org.uk/guidance/ng140/chapter/Recommenda tions. Accessed 24 October 2019.

NMC (Nursing and Midwifery Council) (2019). Revalidation. Your step-by-step guide through the process, http://revalidation.nmc.org.uk. Accessed 13October 2019.

PHE (Public Health England) (2018). MMR (measles, mumps, rubella) vaccine: advice for pregnant women, www.gov.uk/government/publications/vacci ne-in-pregnancy-advice-for-pregnant-women/mmr-measles-mumps-rubella-vaccine-advice-for-pregnant-women.

PHE (Public Health England) (2019). Physical activity for pregnant women, https://assets.publishing.service.gov.uk/government/uploads/system/uploads/ attachment_data/file/829894/5-physical-activity-for-pregnant-women.pdf.

UNICEF (2019) Having meaningful conversations with mothers, www.unicef. org.uk/babyfriendly/wp-content/uploads/sites/2/2018/10/Having-meaning ful-conversations-with-mothers.pdf. Accessed 27 October 2019.

WHO (World Health Organization) (2016). WHO recommendations on antenatal care for a positive pregnancy experience, https://apps.who.int/iris/ bitstream/handle/10665/250796/9789241549912-eng.pdf;jsessionid=9AE3E 1D122FCA29FADA7BDAF31808D69?sequence=1. Accessed 24 October 2019.

WHO (World Health Organization) (2019). Body Mass Index – BMI, www. euro.who.int/en/health-topics/disease-prevention/nutrition/a-healthy-lifes tyle/body-mass-index-bmi. Accessed 11 September 2019.

6

LABOUR AND BIRTH CARE

INTRODUCTION

No two births are the same. A woman's individual social and emotional circumstances, life experiences and physical anatomy will influence the process and outcome of her labour. In addition, the nature of the care she receives can impact on how she perceives the experience, with lasting consequences. In this chapter we will explore how the role of the midwife can be critical to the women achieving the birth experience she aspires to. It begins with an overview of the midwife's role in intrapartum care using the patchwork model (see Figure 6.1) described in Chapter 2.

PROFESSIONAL – ACCOUNTABLE AND SAFE

Above all else, the woman needs to feel that she is in safe hands and that the midwives she meets will provide a high standard of care at all times. When a midwife registers with the Nursing and Midwifery Council (NMC), or other licensing body depending on where she is working, she becomes an accountable practitioner. She should be able to provide a rationale for the actions she takes, having considered the suitable options. Women have their own hopes and expectations for how they want their birth to be, so the midwife needs to be able to discuss the options with women and ensure they know the implications of any choices made.

Women also need to feel psychologically safe. Whilst women in high-income countries have high expectations that they will be

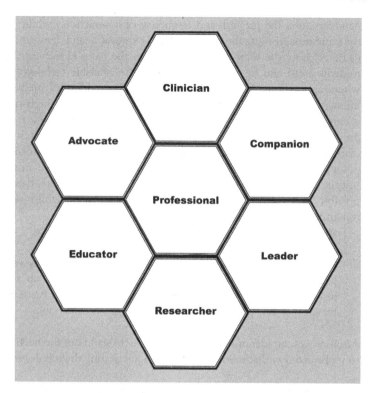

Figure 6.1 The midwife's role: patchwork model

involved in decisions about their care (Molenaar et al. 2018), such aspirations are far from reality for so many women globally. Although the availability of obstetric care is increasing, for many women in low- and middle-income countries (LMICs) the lack of compassion received and potential abuse they face can lead to disengagement and avoidance rather than reduce access to potentially life-saving treatment (Bohren et al. 2014).

CLINICIAN – SKILLED AND COMPETENT

When a woman is in labour the midwife needs to use a range of skills that have taken time to learn and develop. She will be able to use her hands to assess the strength and frequency of contractions, whilst, at the same time, reading the woman's facial expressions and demeanour to detect how the woman is responding to the pain. However, the midwife must also be able to work with the available technology, where appropriate, to monitor and detect when additional medical input might be required. For example, if a woman has a high-risk pregnancy, perhaps because she has developed a condition such as pre-eclampsia, or if she has an underlying medical diagnosis such as diabetes, the midwife must be able to use electronic monitoring equipment, manage a range of intravenous lines, observe urine output and detect deterioration of the fetal heart. Of course, this is possible, but the real test is whether it can be done whilst also remaining calm and adopting a reassuring demeanour.

For example, one woman in the PINK study remembered:

> I was just left to it. The being scared. I was just left to it really. They were just kind of clipping this on and swabbing that, and topping this up, and just working. No kind of, you know, personal contact at all. It was as though they were just working around me to get this done (170).

Another woman identified that for a midwife to stand out she needed to work in a way that involved more than just getting the job done:

> A lot of the midwives I think are very caring. Some of them aren't, but I think it, it doesn't mean they're not doing their job properly. It's that extra something that (pause: 2 seconds) they love what they're doing. And they really genuinely care. It's just the warmth, it's not just coming in, 'Oh, I'm just checking your —' I don't know, it's this warmth from people (laughs slightly). I don't think I could do it (laughs). I just think, some of the midwives, you can just tell they shine, outshine other midwives (171).

COMPANION – COMMUNICATING AND NURTURING

The sense that staff were being open and honest enables women to feel at ease (Baston 2006).

Having access to information is part of the process of making choices and involving women in decisions about their care. It is important, however, that it is pitched at the right level for each woman so that she can make maximum use of it without feeling out of her depth or condescended to. Women have access to a wide range of information, of varying quality and some seek clarification from the midwife. It is essential therefore that they are able to communicate effectively and respect each other's experience.

There were many examples in the PINK study where midwives demonstrated that they cared about the women they had looked after, by going out of their way to continue their contact with them, over and above their usual duties:

> Oh she was lovely. She was really nice. Erm, she actually went off shift, she finished her shift, I think she finished, she finished at six, but she stayed, she didn't go home, she stayed 'til I had [baby] at half past eight and she waited until I had her before she went home [...] it was lovely, it really was, she cared. She didn't just, you know, I wasn't just another pregnant woman in a long line of pregnant women, she actually bothered to stay and see how, what happened (172).

ADVOCATE – PROTECTING AND ENABLING

It was important to women that when staff were not with them that they could be called upon without being made to feel that they were being troublesome. Staff who gave women the impression that they were there for them and not hurrying off to their next job had a rare gift:

> She was kind, efficient, nothing, she, she didn't ever seem tired. Erm, so when I saw her, when she was helping me I didn't ever feel that I was intruding on something she was supposed to be doing, or she was tired with the whole process, which helped. I think sometimes you get staff and they are tired and then you do start to feel almost as if you are bothering them (171).

EDUCATOR – FACILITATING LEARNING

Midwives support women and their families to learn and understand their situation by giving feedback about labour progress and what to expect. It is important that they can gauge when a woman needs more information or when she is overloaded. It can be difficult sometimes for women to visualise what the midwife is talking about when she is talking about the parts of her anatomy she cannot see. Midwives often use analogies to provide a more understandable depiction of a situation. For example, she could explain how initially her cervix felt firm like the tip of a nose but now it has softened and feels more like lips. When describing to a woman how her cervix is dilating and how the contractions have helped this process, the midwife might say that the neck of the womb was long like the neck of a polo neck jumper but now its length has been taken up into the body of the uterus and the cervix is open like a crew neck.

Often midwives are looking after student midwives too. As the midwife explains what she is doing to her apprentice, she is also giving important information to the woman and her partner. Helping women understand what is happening to them is a valuable exercise in helping her feel more in control and part of the decision-making process. Shared decision-making between parents and professionals is associated with greater satisfaction for both parties (Molenaar et al. 2018).

RESEARCHER – CREATOR OF NEW KNOWLEDGE

There are many aspects of labour care that there is still no evidence for, often because it would be inappropriate to undertake a randomised controlled trial (RCT) to establish causality. For example, it would be unethical to randomise women to receive care in a particular location for many reasons, as identified in a pilot study in the Netherlands asking women about their willingness to take part in an RCT regarding homebirth versus home-like short-stay hospital birth (Hendrix et al. 2009). Women are encouraged to exercise choice throughout pregnancy and childbirth hence the thought of having a decision made for them, through randomisation, is not always palatable or, indeed, wholly understood.

Midwives must therefore work with researchers, or become researchers, in order to understand and overcome the complexities of recruiting women to research studies and generate new knowledge to feedback into maternity care, and ironically ultimately giving more choice to women. Investment in clinician-led research globally would increase ownership and buy-in regarding the value of local research; whilst much evidence is transferable some practices require a culturally and facility-specific investigation in order for it to be applied in practice (Dye et al. 2013).

LEADER – CHANGE AGENT

To be able to make changes in clinical environments, midwives need to have a comprehensive understanding of contemporary working practices. They need to understand the staff and walk in the shoes of those who have been accustomed to providing care in a particular way. Inevitably, with change comes a degree of uncertainty, and midwives need to have the courage to drive change where it has the potential to enhance the care of women and working conditions. Such midwifery leaders also need support from their senior colleagues with the recognition that successful practice developments depend on how well the workforce copes with the unknown (Russell 2018). Staff need to be involved and consulted in any proposed changes, understand the rationale behind them and have opportunities for appropriate skills acquisition to be able to move forward.

The midwife must regularly show leadership when caring for women in labour. For example, this might be in relation to having the courage to challenge a senior professional's decision. The midwife must represent the woman's best interests when there is a difficult situation. One woman in the PINK study recognised the intervention of her midwife which resulted in swift remedial action; she said:

> Dr wanted me to have a natural birth. The midwife was so concerned she advised her supervisor and the consultant was called. Within a short time, I had an emergency caesarean section as the baby was in distress (162).

Thus, the interventions made by midwives on a daily basis can be life-saving and have far-reaching implications for those in their care.

SO, WHAT IS INTRAPARTUM CARE?

The International Confederation of Midwives (ICM) essential competencies for midwifery practice (ICM 2018) categorises labour care into:

1 Promote physiologic labour and birth
2 Manage a safe spontaneous vaginal birth and prevent complications
3 Provide care of the newborn immediately after birth

These global competencies will be used throughout the chapter to provide a framework to describe the role of the midwife in intrapartum care. They should be considered in light of growing global recognition that women's experience of care is important; that it's not just what we do but the way that we do it that matters to women (Tuncalp et al. 2015).

PROMOTE PHYSIOLOGIC LABOUR AND BIRTH

PROVIDE CARE FOR A WOMAN IN THE BIRTH SETTING OF HER CHOICE

In the UK, women are offered choice regarding where they give birth, subject to where is considered the safest option for them and what options are available. That said, some women prefer a particular option, irrespective of her risk status; for example, she may wish for a home birth even though she has a scar on her uterus from a previous caesarean section. The role of the midwife is to give the woman evidence-based information, ensure she understands it and then support the woman in her choice. The midwife may ask for support from senior colleagues if she feels that the woman may be putting herself in danger; it is always appropriate to run concerns past a colleague to ensure that nothing has been missed, or to consider if a compromise could be found.

OBTAIN RELEVANT OBSTETRIC AND MEDICAL HISTORY

If the woman has been accessing antenatal care, her previous obstetric and medical history will be well documented, either in a hand-held record or digitally. When the woman is attended in labour, be it at home or maternity unit, her pregnancy history should also be reviewed, to identify any changes or cause for concern. Then her current health and reason why she had made contact today should be discussed and recorded. If the woman has a birth plan this should be read together with the woman and any changes to it identified.

The midwife then assesses the woman's current state of health by performing routine observations of temperature, pulse and blood pressure and urinalysis. The length, strength and frequency of contractions is observed, along with how the woman is responding to them. The uterus is palpated to assess the growth, lie and presentation of the fetus, as well as estimating engagement of the presenting part in the woman's pelvis. The midwife asks about fetal movements and auscultates the fetal heart, usually via a doppler so that the woman and her birth partner can hear it. The midwife recognises that the heart rate should be between 110–160 beats per minute (NICE 2014).

If the woman has been well during her pregnancy and she has not been anaemic, there are no indications to request any laboratory tests. However, if she has previously been treated for anaemia and there is no recent full blood count result to see if she has responded to treatment, the midwife will take blood to determine her haemoglobin levels. For a woman who is at risk of having an operative birth, for example if she has had a previous caesarean, blood will be taken for blood grouping in preparation for the unlikely event that she may need a transfusion.

The labour and birth process is traditionally characterised by three apparently distinct phases.

The first stage of labour begins with a latent phase, during which time the cervix begins to soften, shorten and dilate. Uterine contractions are often irregular and short lived during this phase but can be uncomfortable and distressing to the woman, particularly if she is told that despite her pain, that her cervix remains closed. Maternity professionals deem that the first stage of labour has not truly become established until the cervix is thin and 4 cm dilated.

Once this milestone has been reached, labour is recognised as having begun its trajectory towards the inevitable birth and with this recognition also comes a change in its monitoring and supervision.

During labour and birth, women need feedback about their progress and fetal well-being. They need to know about routine observations and when they will be made. Not explaining what to expect can leave women feeling vulnerable and out of control. Women experiencing labour and birth need information and one woman in the PINK study (Baston 2006) commented that childbirth is an everyday event for midwives. She urged midwives:

> Just try and realise that this one person might actually be quite scared, and not really know what's happening, and just keep reassuring them and telling them what is happening as much as possible (173).

Birth partners also need to be kept informed and be encouraged that the support they are providing is so valuable to their partner. The woman will pick up on subtleties, any collusion between the partner and midwife; she needs to be able to trust in their unswerving support for her efforts. Labour and birth can be a long process and the midwife may come to the end of her shift before the woman has her baby. When this happens, the midwife can help alleviate any trepidation the woman has about being cared for by someone new, by introducing her in a positive manner.

PROVIDE RESPECTFUL ONE-TO-ONE CARE

It is important that the woman feels involved in decisions about her care; her wishes should be considered at all times. Her dignity and privacy should be central to midwifery care and the midwife should ensure that she respects her personal space by knocking and waiting before she enters her room. The woman's permission should be sought before all procedures, even if this means waiting until an appropriate moment to discuss something with her. It is an expectation in the UK that once a woman is in established labour, she has access to one-to-one care from her midwife. In reality on a busy labour ward, a midwife may be caring for another woman at the same time. However, if that is the case, both women should not be in the active phase of labour as this would preclude appropriate one-to-one care for both. If the midwife needs to leave the room, she should explain when she will be back and ensure both the woman and her birth partner know how to summon help in her absence.

ENCOURAGE FREEDOM OF MOVEMENT AND UPRIGHT POSITIONS

Women feel more in control when they are upright and freedom of movement and mobility facilitate labour progress and comfort. There are many ways that the midwife can facilitate an active labour, which can work as a distraction technique as well as passing time. Many modern labour wards have a range of soft furnishings and bespoke birthing aids, such as balls, mats and kneeling stools, to help the woman stay upright. Sometimes women need permission and encouragement to get off the bed; rooms where the bed is not central in the room can help convey the message that it is not considered a mandatory piece of equipment.

PROVIDE NOURISHMENT AND FLUIDS

The midwife will encourage the woman to drink to her thirst during labour, and isotonic drinks may provide extra salts and calories when a woman does not feel like snacking. Labour is hard and hot work, offering frequent sips of iced water to the labouring woman is a job that the birth partner can be encouraged to do. Women who are well and who are not expected to need a general anaesthetic, or have not received opioids in labour, can eat a light diet during labour if they wish (NICE 2014).

OFFER AND SUPPORT WOMAN TO USE STRATEGIES FOR COPING WITH LABOUR PAIN

If the woman has made a birth plan it is likely that she has provided some detail about how she would like to manage her labour pain. This plan can be reviewed as and when circumstances change. For example, if the woman did not want to have any pharmaceutical pain relief, but then events require that she has her labour augmented, she may then want to consider other options to help her with the imposition of induced contractions. Alternatively, women may plan to have an epidural from the outset, as did 'Rachel' in the PINK study:

> I decided on my birth plan that I wanted an epidural [...] I'm not one of these people who want to go back to the cave man days and erm do everything without pain relief. Erm, I wanted it to be a positive experience and that meant pain-free for me [...] Absolutely crystal clear that I wanted an epidural (76).

She remained adamant that she did not want to experience a painful labour:

> And erh, I remember when I went into the labour suite, the, the midwife on duty said, 'Ohh, would you like a lavender bath?' and I said, 'No I want drugs!' (laughs) 'I do not want a lavender bath!' (76)

The power of contractions and the need to delve deep to find the strength to endure them means that some women feel like they are in another world. Not all women are able to articulate how they are feeling. One woman in the PINK study said:

> My husband said that I didn't make any noise at all but inside my head I was screaming very loudly. Possibly I should have done it out loud – why I didn't I don't know (85).

Conversely, some women use their voices as a means of release, and may moan, groan, shout, scream and sometimes swear, throughout labour. The midwife needs to be able to know the difference between distress and this natural coping mechanism, and also reassure the birth partner that noise is fine.

Going through labour without any drugs is a huge achievement, and women who want this and attain this experience an amazing sense of accomplishment that transcends into many other areas of their life. Helping a woman achieve her goals is also extremely satisfying for midwives and they often say and feel that they have been on that journey too. It takes intense effort to help a woman breathe through each and every contraction and to be by her side coaching her through when she feels like she cannot continue, but the rewards are immeasurable when the woman is beaming with joy as she holds her new baby. The use of water to relieve labour pain is growing in popularity, and along with playing the music of her choice can lead to a joyful experience, as this senior midwife recounts:

> A memorable occasion (of many) was when a woman came onto labour ward obviously in labour with her sister-in-law as a birth partner. The woman was from Thailand and her sister-in-law was from Poland. I thought the sister-in-law could speak Thai because they were chattering away together and giggling. As it turned out they could not speak each other's languages or English but it did not seem to matter. I used a telephone interpreter for decision making but for most of the time we three managed a rather successful sign language. The women wanted music and so we had music (polish polka tunes), we danced, we laughed the woman had a beautiful relaxed birth leaning over the bed, giggling and swinging her hips between pushes. My student was amazed. I remember this because it was a room full of joy. The communication between us was powerful although not in the usual manner and the resulting experience was good for all of us. I learnt that birth does not have to be sombre.
>
> Adele Stanley, midwifery-led unit lead midwife, UK

Sometime the best laid plans are not always realised and sometime the position of the baby or untoward events means that the woman needs to accept an epidural in order to get through the rest of the labour. The midwife has an important role in ensuring that the woman feels supported in her decision, that she understands what the procedure will involve and above all does not feel that she has failed because of it.

ASSESS REGULARLY PARAMETERS OF MATERNAL–FETAL STATUS

The midwife continues to observe the woman's vital signs throughout labour, in line with evidence-based guidance (NICE 2014). She listens to the fetal heart and monitors the frequency, strength and length of contractions, any fluid lost and what methods the woman is using to cope with her pain.

The main focus of these assessments is that the woman and her baby are tolerating labour well and making progress towards birth.

Before labour starts and in the last few weeks of pregnancy, the cervix changes from being firm and posterior and difficult to reach, to softening (ripening) and becoming more central. As noted in Chapter 1, the cervix further effaces and dilates during labour and the subtle changes can be detected by the midwife during a vaginal examination (VE). This provides valuable feedback to both the woman and her carer, that the contractions are doing their job, that the cervix is opening and the baby is descending.

Whilst women do want feedback about their progress, vaginal examination can be a distressing or uncomfortable procedure. It is important that a VE is necessary and this intimate assessment is therefore not usually performed more than every four hours in an uncomplicated labour. Vaginal examinations can be a potential avenue for introducing infection, especially if the membranes are no longer intact, therefore their use should be minimal and judicial.

The midwife becomes skilled at 'measuring' dilatation by what she can feel with the two gloved fingers she is using to gently assess the cervix. For example, when the cervix is 3 cm dilated, the midwife can insert two closed fingers. The length of the cervix is also assessed as well as how well the fetal head is applied to it. During this examination the decent of the head is also noted and this is described as the 'station'. Further detail is discerned when the midwife can actually feel the bones on the fetal head and, from identifying key landmarks, determine which way the baby is facing. If the membranes are still intact, the midwife will usually feel a bag of forewaters, depending on how well applied the head is to the cervix.

Some women decline VEs, and their wishes should be respected. All women need information in order to make the decision that is right for their individual circumstances. In an urgent situation, for example if there was sudden fetal distress in labour, it is usual practice to undertake a VE to determine if the cervix is fully dilated. Women should be aware that the purpose of this would be to see if there is the option of delivering the baby by forceps or ventouse, rather than resorting to a caesarean which would be needed if the cervix was still dilating. In such circumstances, the woman might be willing to have a VE, but still decline 'routine' examinations.

USE LABOUR PROGRESS GRAPHIC DISPLAY TO RECORD FINDINGS

The routine use of a partogram, a single pre-printed sheet to document progress in labour in graphic form, is contentious. Based on the documentation of cervical dilatation in 100 primigravida at term, the Friedman curve was developed to identify 'normal' progress in labour (Friedman 1954). Deviation from the curve is used to highlight when action should take place to expedite the birth because of lack of progress. An alert line represents labour progress in the slowest 10 per cent of women, and the action line is set at two or four hours after that (Lavender et al. 2012). NICE (2014) guidance recommends the use of a partogram with a four-hour action line. The partogram is also used to record other maternal and fetal observations, such as blood pressure and the fetal heart rate, and therefore provides an overview of the history of a woman's labour, which is particularly valuable when care is handed over to another midwife.

PREVENT UNNECESSARY ROUTINE INTERVENTIONS

As the advocate for woman and facilitator of spontaneous birth, the midwife aims to avoid the use of interventions that are not evidence based. There are many interventions that were routinely practised in the belief that they had a beneficial impact on maternal health. For example, in the past, it was believed that routine episiotomy would protect the woman from severe vaginal trauma; however, systematic reviews of the evidence has now disputed the efficacy of such practice, as it does not reduce perineal pain, incontinence or painful intercourse (Jiang et al. 2017).

Globally, however, not all women have the benefit of receiving high-quality midwifery care. Whilst it is clearly important not to intervene unnecessarily for clinical reasons, it is equally important that women feel safe to access care and do not fear that their birth attendant will perform such techniques without a justified rationale. In countries where place of birth is transitioning to facility provision and a medicalised ethos, some women are at risk of being subject to interventions without their consent. Such 'obstetric violence' is more prevalent in contexts where women are poor and oppressed (Perera et al. 2018). In efforts to protect women from degrading and disrespectful care globally, the World Health Organization (WHO 2018) makes recommendations for care that enhances a woman's experience, recognising the importance of respect and kindness provided by skilled midwives.

AUGMENT UTERINE CONTRACTILITY JUDICIOUSLY

Delay in the first stage of labour is usually suspected if cervical dilatation is less than 2 cm in four hours when the woman is in the established labour (NICE 2014). The midwife has a role in trying to prevent such delay by ensuring that the woman is hydrated, supported and has one-to-one care. Amniotomy (ARM) may be considered and discussed with the woman where progress is slow and the membranes are intact. The midwife should explain that whilst the length of labour may be reduced, she may experience more painful contractions and other options for pain relief should be thought through. If delay is confirmed, the midwife should refer the woman to the care of an obstetrician who will undertake a full assessment of her progress before considering intervention, such as the use of intravenous oxytocin.

MANAGE A SAFE SPONTANEOUS VAGINAL BIRTH AND PREVENT COMPLICATIONS

SUPPORT THE WOMAN TO GIVE BIRTH IN HER POSITION OF CHOICE

Gone are the days when women were expected to adopt the position that best suited the accoucheur (person assisting child-birth); midwives of today need to be agile and able to support a woman adopt whatever position she finds comfortable. Often birth positions can be influenced by the layout of the room, therefore it is important that the furniture is arranged to facilitate mobility and upright positions where possible and that the bed is not centre stage. Sometimes the woman becomes fixed in a particular position and may need gentle encouragement by the midwife to move around, particularly if the contractions have become less frequent.

COACH WOMAN ABOUT PUSHING TO CONTROL EXPULSION OF PRESENTING PART

When the woman is in the second stage of labour she may instinctively have the urge to push. There has been much debate about the way that women are coached to push; either closed glottis, where the woman takes a deep breath and holds it while she pushes, or a more flexible and responsive approach. Much will depend on if she is making progress and the presenting part is advancing. Whilst ever she and the baby are well and there are no signs of distress, she should be encouraged to work with her body. If she has an epidural, however, she will usually require some instruction and feedback about when a contraction is coming, so that she can work with the expulsive efforts of the uterus.

UNDERTAKE APPROPRIATE MANOEUVRES AND USE MATERNAL POSITION TO FACILITATE BIRTH

In most situations, birth is a spontaneous event which requires only the patience and watchful waiting of the midwife. When all is progressing well, the midwife observes the head advancing and gives the woman feedback about how events are progressing. As the head is crowning, the midwife encourages the woman to refrain from active pushing and to gently breathe the head out, to reduce the likelihood of trauma to the pelvic floor. There is debate about whether the midwife should actively apply pressure to the fetal head to keep it flexed with the aim of facilitating its slower emergence, or to have her hands poised just in case it suddenly advances and needs restraint. In the event, the midwife will judge each situation depending on how engaged the mother is, how quickly the head is advancing.

Once the head is born, the shoulders usually follow with the next contraction, one at a time. They may emerge spontaneously or be facilitated by the midwife applying gentle traction on the head to guide the birth of the rest of the baby's body. The midwife has a detailed understanding of the mechanism of birth and can help facilitate safe delivery when the baby's position is not straightforward, such as in a face or posterior presentation. She is also trained to expedite the birth if the baby is in a breech position.

EXPEDITE BIRTH IN PRESENCE OF FETAL DISTRESS

If there are signs that the baby is distressed, the midwife needs to engage the woman with active pushing if birth is imminent. If, however, there is no advancement of the fetal head and the baby is distressed, the midwife will summon the support of an obstetrician who may decide that an instrumental birth (forceps or vacuum) is the best option. Occasionally, an episiotomy, performed with informed consent and analgesia, may provide sufficient room for the head to advance and birth to be facilitated. However, if the woman is not in second stage when distress is diagnosed, the safest option may be caesarean section. It is particularly important that the midwife maintains a calm and relaxed demeanour and keeps the woman and her partner informed of her actions. One woman in the PINK study recalls how much she valued the calm manner in which she was prepared to go to theatre:

> I think just, the fact that it was, it was all so normal and they weren't rushing about – you know like you see on ER and Casualty and Holby, there was none of that urgency, none of that 'oh my God, we've got to get this baby out, you know or else the world is going to end!' It was all perfectly normal, perfectly friendly (174).

Most women readily accept modifications to their plans when faced with a clinical situation where their ideas need to change; choice becomes a lesser outcome when faced with potential fetal compromise (Armstrong & Kenyon 2017). However, involvement in decisions should continue to be the default position as it is associated with a positive appraisal of the birth.

DELAY CORD CLAMPING

It has been routine practice in obstetric care to clamp and cut the cord immediately after the birth of the baby. However, research has now shown that by facilitating delayed cord clamping (DCC) and leaving the cord intact for at least one minute, the baby receives more blood from the placenta. This practice leads to an increased red blood cell count, which is particularly important if the baby is premature or in a LMIC where iron-rich foods and recourse to blood transfusions is less readily available (WHO 2014). The evidence continues to grow in this area; a recent RCT study (Mercer et al. 2018) demonstrated greater ferritin levels in babies who received DCC, which led to increased brain myelination at four months of age.

ASSESS IMMEDIATE CONDITION OF NEWBORN

Thankfully most babies take a deep breath in soon after birth and cry, enabling the parents and midwife to also take a sigh of relief. Sometimes babies are slower to cry and gentle stimulation with a warm dry towel is all that is required to prompt it to breathe. The midwife is watching carefully as the baby is being born for a range of characteristics that reassure her that all is well. Importantly the baby should have a good tone and be centrally pink in colour, although its extremities may be blue and its face congested if second stage has been prolonged. After one minute of age the midwife uses a scoring system, called the Apgar score, to assess well-being and this is performed again at five minutes. The score includes observations of tone, colour, heart rate, breathing and responsiveness.

PROVIDE SKIN-TO-SKIN CONTACT AND WARM ENVIRONMENT

In the last few decades in the UK, we have gone from 'delivering' the baby, examining, weighing and then swaddling it before handing it back to its mother like a parcel, towards immediate skin-to-skin contact between mother and baby at birth. This close experience is now more of an expectation of all women than a choice by the well informed. This movement is borne from increasing evidence of the benefits of skin-to-skin contact, not just at birth or with full-term infants, but as a healing and nurturing experience for both parents at any time.

All women should have the opportunity to hold their new baby in skin-to-skin contact soon after birth, even if birth takes place in theatre (Brodrick & Baston 2017). It has many known benefits, including keeping the baby warm, regulating its respirations and calming the mother. Skin-to-skin contact is also known to facilitate breastfeeding especially when uninterrupted. Women should be offered skin-to-skin contact with their baby irrespective of how they intend to feed their baby and wherever their baby is born

(UNICEF 2019). For more information on how the midwife supports breastfeeding, see Chapter 7.

DELIVER PLACENTA AND MEMBRANES AND INSPECT FOR COMPLETENESS

The woman should have had the opportunity to consider, antenatally, how she would like the placenta to be delivered. It has been common obstetric practice to offer an injection of a synthetic oxytocin as this reduces the length of third stage thereby reducing the risk of bleeding. However, there are side effects to this drug and sometimes women feel sick, etc. If progress in labour has been uneventful and there are no contraindications, such as previous haemorrhage, then a physiological third stage can be awaited. This takes about 15 minutes although it can take up to one hour (Baston & Hall 2017). The midwife awaits signs of separation of the placenta from the uterine wall and she can palpate that the uterus has contracted and then encourage the woman to gently push the placenta out. It is an important role of the midwife to inspect the placenta after the birth to ensure it is complete and that there are no cotyledons left behind which could prevent the uterus from contracting efficiently and also be a potential source of infection.

ASSESS UTERINE TONE, MAINTAIN FIRM CONTRACTION AND ESTIMATE AND RECORD MATERNAL

The tone of the uterus immediately after birth should be very firm and this is a reassuring feature which the midwife palpates abdominally. The uterus should be central and not deviated by a full bladder. The midwife also estimates how much blood the woman has lost and records this on the partogram along with the woman's postnatal blood pressure, temperature and pulse. If there are signs of ongoing bleeding the midwife will review the contraction of the uterus and manually stimulate it to contract if it has relaxed; she may consider giving an injection of oxytocin to induce and sustain contraction.

INSPECT VAGINAL AND PERINEAL AREAS FOR TRAUMA, AND REPAIR AS NEEDED

The midwife then examines the woman's genital tract for any trauma that might have occurred. She may have observed the perineum tearing during the birth or it may have appeared intact, yet there may be tearing to the vaginal wall which needs suturing. This inspection is not pleasant for the woman and she may wish to have some gas and air or focus on her baby while the midwife assesses the perineum. The midwife needs to be gentle and efficient in this examination, so that the woman can then relax and enjoy her baby. If suturing is needed, the midwife can undertake this procedure if she has had additional training and achieved the required competence. The midwife will use a continuous, dissolvable, subcuticular suture to the skin as this has been shown to be the most comfortable for women (NICE 2014).

PROVIDE CARE OF THE NEWBORN IMMEDIATELY AFTER BIRTH

Unless a concern has been identified before the baby is born, it should be given to the mother straightaway and placed in skin-to-skin contact. Whilst on its mother's abdomen the midwife will dry the baby with a warm towel and then cover with a fresh dry towel and put a hat on him so that he does not lose heat by evaporation. It is extremely important that the baby does not drop its temperature and for this reason, birthing rooms are kept warm and draught free.

If the baby does not breathe spontaneously, the midwife will continue to stimulate him by rubbing with the towel, talking to him and reassuring the parents. During this time, the cord should remain intact so that the baby is benefiting from the blood pulsating down the cord. The midwife will consider the whole picture when assessing the baby's well-being: has the mother had medication in labour, was there any fetal distress, what is the baby's tone and colour? She will listen to the baby's heart rate and use all of these parameters to decide what action to take next. Midwives receive mandatory annual updates in neonatal and maternal resuscitation and can commence life-saving resuscitation until neonatal staff arrive, if further assistance is required.

The first hour after birth is often described as the golden hour (Crenshaw 2014), during which time the new parents and the baby are getting to know each other and are exploring each other's faces. As we know and learn more about the instinctive behaviours of the newborn we can allow nature to kick in and for the baby to make its own way to the breast, rather than assist it to feed as often happened previously. Levels of oxytocin are running high in both the other and the baby immediately after birth; the effect on the mother is to tune into her baby and want to nurture and nourish him. Oxytocin also assists in the ejection of her milk, and the first milk colostrum will be readily available for her baby at this time.

CONDUCT A COMPLETE PHYSICAL EXAMINATION OF NEWBORN IN PRESENCE OF THE PARENTS

The midwife undertakes the first top-to-toe examination of the baby in the first hour after birth. Most of this can be done while the mother holds her baby in skin-to-skin contact and completed when the baby makes its obligatory trip to the weighing scales and photo shoot. It is a comprehensive check to ensure there are no major physical abnormalities, including examination of the palate, counting digits and ensuring the spine is intact and the anus is patent.

Whilst the baby remains in skin-to-skin contact, consent will be sought to administer vitamin K to the baby as this reduces the risk of Vitamin K Deficiency Bleeding (previously known as haemorrhagic disease of the newborn), which is a life-threatening condition that babies are at particular risk of if the birth has been traumatic. Rather than testing babies for it, vitamin K is routinely offered to all (NICE 2006). The baby should ideally be left in skin-to-skin contact until it has its first feed, breast or formula. Both parents should be shown how to support and hold their baby safely, ensuring that the face is visible at all times and the head and neck are in a neutral position so as not to occlude the airway.

THE ROLE OF THE MIDWIFE IN COMPLICATED BIRTH

There is much emphasis on the fact that midwives are experts in the practice and protection of normal birth. However, they continue to care for women whose birth is facilitated by operative means and are the key person who has usually been with them throughout labour and can therefore provide a reassuring face and voice, when other professionals come into the room to assist with the birth. Women might require assistance for a range of reasons including: fetal compromise, fetal position, fetal presentation, cord prolapse, bleeding, hypertension and lack of labour progress. The advocacy role of the midwife is particularly important at this time; she knows what the woman had wished for and can ensure that as many of her aspirations are upheld as possible.

Depending on local policy, midwives will usually continue to care for the woman, by preparing her for surgery, including ensuring she is catheterised, so that the bladder is not damaged during the operation. She will assist the woman to change into a theatre gown, take off any jewellery and put on anti-embolic stocking to reduce the risk of thrombosis. The midwife will then change into theatre scrubs, show the birth partner where to do the same, and accompany the woman, supporting her during the insertion of a regional anaesthetic. Many large units have bespoke theatre teams comprising operating theatre practitioners, a support worker and scrub nurses. There will be two obstetricians to perform the surgery and an anaesthetist to monitor the maternal condition throughout. The midwife will listen to the fetal heart prior to commencement of the operation and then be responsible for caring for the baby once born. If there is any suspicion that the baby will be compromised at birth, there will also be a neontologist or neonatal nurse practitioner present.

Abdominal surgery generally carries the potential life-threatening risks of anaesthetic complications, haemorrhage, thromboembolism and infection, and caesarean section is no exception. However, the increased prevalence of caesarean birth means that it is a common mode of birth and one that some women choose rather than to opt for a vaginal birth. When labour ends in caesarean birth, however, women can be left with a range of emotions; emergency caesarean birth was associated with a negative perception of the birth compared with elective caesarean and vaginal birth (Baston 2006).

Women sometimes feel that they missed out on the visual as well as the physical aspects of the baby being born. In the PINK study, one woman describes that she had no idea what the caesarean involved, in terms of the surgical procedure and what was done to her body.

> I haven't seen a caesarean section on, on television on medical programmes, and I would love to, because I have no idea what they did, what they did to me, 'cos they'd got a bl, a sheet up. I would love to see, erm, I'd love to see what the experience is. But I've no idea (77).

In some units, the obstetrician lowers the drapes that screen the woman from seeing the operation field, enabling the woman to see her baby as soon as it is born. One woman in the PINK study was saddened by her separation from the baby at birth:

> I was a bit disappointed, 'cos I'd seen on telly people having caesarean, and they had given the baby to the woman, to hold herself, but they didn't offer him to me, they gave him to my husband [...] I was very disappointed that I couldn't hold him myself, Erm, but, they then went and put him in a cot, erm and put him in another room, and sent my husband through to that room (193).

Babies born by caesarean are more likely to have complications at birth but the majority of these will relate to the indication for caesarean rather than to the surgery itself. There are some potential risks, however, including laceration during surgery and transient tachypnoea of the newborn (Baston & Durward 2017). There is some evidence that women who have a planned caesarean are less likely to intend to breastfeed and more likely to stop breastfeeding than other women (Hobbs et al. 2016). The same study found that women who had an emergency caesarean were more likely to experience breastfeeding difficulties. Midwives have an important role in supporting women who have a surgical birth to benefit from skin-to-skin contact, to receive adequate pain relief and support to find comfortable positions to feed and care for their babies.

CONCLUSION

The midwife is the lead professional for labour and birth care in low-risk pregnancies. She plays an important role in ensuring that the woman and her partner have a positive experience irrespective of where or how birth takes place. She provides safe, accountable, evidence-based care involving the woman in decision-making throughout. Birth can be a transformative experience for all involved. Midwives need to be able to adapt their approach to the woman in front of them and her unique circumstances, fears and aspirations. Showing kindness and compassion can help women cope with the hard work that labour requires.

RESOURCES

Baston H, and Hall J (2017). *Labour*. 2nd ed. Midwifery essentials, volume 3. Edinburgh: Elsevier. This is a comprehensive handbook with chapters covering all stages of labour, pain relief, induction of labour, caesarean birth and perineal repair.

Johnson R, and Taylor W (2016). *Skills for midwifery practice*. 4th ed. Oxford: Elsevier Health Science.

NHS Choices (2019), www.nhs.uk/conditions/pregnancy-and-ba by/how-to-make-birth-plan/. How to make a birth plan. This article covers what to include and consider when preparing for birth.

Redshaw M, Martin C, Savage-Glynn E, and Harrison S (2019). Women's experiences of maternity care in England: preliminary development of a standard measure. *BMC Pregnancy and Childbirth* 19:167, https://bmcpregnancychildbirth.biomedcentral.com/articles/10.1186/s12884-019-2284-9.

Royal College of Obstetricians and Gynaecologists (2015). Reducing the risk of thromboembolism during pregnancy and the puerperium. Green Top Guideline No. 37a, https://www.rcog.org.uk/globalassets/documents/guidelines/gtg-37a.pdf.

Tommy's (2019) 5 positive ways to prepare for labour, www.tomm ys.org/pregnancy-information/labour-birth/5-positive-ways-prepare-labour. This valuable resource has a range of additional vignettes about issues such as latent phase of labour, hypnobirthing and birth positions.

UNICEF (2019). Breastfeeding resources, www.unicef.org.uk/ba byfriendly/baby-friendly-resources/breastfeeding-resources/. These resources cover a range of issues around establishing and continuing successful breastfeeding, including videos on positioning and attaching the baby at the breast and meeting baby for the first time. Babies held in uninterrupted skin-to-skin go through nine stages of instinctive behaviour, www.unicef.org.uk/babyfriendly/baby-friendly-resources/rela tionship-building-resources/meeting-baby-for-the-first-time-video/.

REFERENCES

Armstrong N, and Kenyon S (2017). When choice becomes limited: women's experiences of delay in labour. *Health* 21(2):223–238.

Baston H (2006). Women's experience of emergency caesarean birth. PhD thesis. University of York, http://etheses.whiterose.ac.uk/14082/.

Baston H, and Durward H (2017). *Examination of the newborn: a practical guide.* 3rd ed. London: Routledge.

Baston H, and Hall J (2017). *Labour.* 2nd ed. Midwifery essentials, volume 3. Edinburgh: Elsevier.

Bohren M, Hunter E, Munthe-Kaas H, *et al.* (2014). Facilitators and barriers to facility-based delivery in low- and middle-income countries: a qualitative evidence synthesis. *Reprod Health* 11(1):71.

Brodrick A, and Baston H (2017). Taking the drama out of obstetric theatre: implementing change. *MIDIRS Midwifery Digest* 27(4):467–472.

Crenshaw J (2014). Healthy birth practice #6: keep mother and baby together – it's best for mother, baby, and breastfeeding. *The Journal of Perinatal Education* 23(4):211–217.

Dye C, Boerma T, Evans D, *et al.* (2013). The World Health Report 2013: research for universal health coverage. Geneva: World Health Organization, https://apps.who.int/iris/bitstream/handle/10665/85761/9789240690837_eng.pdf?sequence=2. Accessed 1 November 2019.

Friedman E (1954). Graphic analysis of labour. *American Journal of Obstetrics and Gynecology* 68:1568–1575.

Hendrix M, Van Horck M, Moreta F, *et al.* (2009). Why women do not accept randomisation for place of birth: feasibility of a RCT in the Netherlands. *BJOG* 116:549–566.

Hobbs A, Mannion C, and McDonald S (2016). The impact of caesarean section on breastfeeding initiation, duration and difficulties in the first four months postpartum. *BMC Pregnancy and Childbirth* 16, doi:10.1186/s12884-016-0876-1.

ICM (2018). Essential competencies for midwifery practice, www.internationalmidwives.org/assets/files/general-files/2019/03/icm-competencies-en-screens.pdf.

Jiang H, Qian X, Carroli G, *et al.* (2017). Selective versus routine use of episiotomy for vaginal birth. *Cochrane Database of Systematic Reviews* (2), doi:10.1002/14651858.CD000081.pub3.

Lavender T, Hart A, and Smyth RM (2012). Effect of partogram use on outcomes for women in spontaneous labour at term. *Cochrane Database Systematic Reviews* 8(8), doi:10.1002/14651858.CD005461.pub3.

Mercer J, Erickson-Owens D, Deoni S, *et al.* (2018). Effects of delayed cord clamping on 4-month ferritin levels, brain myelin content, and neurodevelopment: a randomized controlled trial. *The Journal of Pediatrics* 203:266–272.

Molenaar J, Korstjens I, Hendrix M, *et al.* (2018). Needs of parents and professionals to improve shared decision-making in interprofessional maternity care practice: a qualitative study. *Birth* 45(3):245–254.

NICE (National Institute for Health and Care Excellence) (2006, updated 2015). Postnatal care up to 8 weeks after birth. NICE CG37, www.nice.org.uk/guidance/cg37. Accessed 1 November 2019.

NICE (National Institute for Health and Care Excellence) (2014, updated 2017). Intrapartum care: care for healthy women and babies. NICE CG190, www.nice.org.uk/guidance/cg190. Accessed 27 October 2019.

Perera D, Lund R, Swahnberg K, *et al.* (2018). 'When helpers hurt': women's and midwives' stories of obstetric violence in state health institutions, Colombo district, Sri Lanka. *BMC Pregnancy and Childbirth* 18, doi:10.1186/s12884-018-1869-z.

Russell K (2018). Factors that support change in the delivery of midwifery led care in hospital settings. a review of current literature. *Women and Birth* 31 (2):E134–141.

Tuncalp O, Were W, MacLennan C, *et al.* (2015). Quality of care for pregnant women and newborns – the WHO vision. *BJOG* 122(8):1045–1049.

UNICEF (2019). Having meaningful conversations with mothers, www.unicef.org.uk/babyfriendly/wp-content/uploads/sites/2/2018/10/Having-meaningful-conversations-with-mothers.pdf. Accessed 27 October 2019.

WHO (World Health Organization) (2014). Guideline: delayed umbilical cord clamping for improved maternal and infant health and nutrition outcomes. Geneva: World Health Organization, https://apps.who.int/iris/bitstream/handle/10665/148793/?sequence=1. Accessed 1 November 2019.

WHO (World Health Organization) (2018). WHO recommendation on episiotomy, https://extranet.who.int/rhl/topics/preconception-pregnancy-childbirth-and-postpartum-care/care-during-childbirth/care-during-labour-2nd-stage/who-recommendation-episiotomy-policy-0.

7

POSTNATAL CARE

INTRODUCTION

The postnatal period, from delivery of the placental to six weeks after the birth, is a precious time during which new parents continue the transition to parenthood and get to know their baby. It is also a time when parents have a sudden realisation of the dependency of the new infant, and with that, the huge responsibility to keep it safe. The midwife has a key part to play in helping protect this special time, enabling the parents to master their new role. It is therefore essential that care is planned with the mother to ensure it is personal to her and helps her achieve her hopes and expectations. This chapter will outline some of the key elements of postnatal care and consider the midwife's role in supporting them. It will therefore include how the midwife can support a mother to develop a close and loving relationship with her baby. It begins with an overview of the midwife's role in postnatal care using the patchwork model (see Figure 7.1) described in Chapter 2.

PROFESSIONAL – ACCOUNTABLE AND SAFE

The midwife caring for women in the postnatal period continues in her remit of being responsible for the care of both the woman and her baby, whilst supporting the family unit to flourish. In the UK, national guidelines (NICE 2006) provide a framework for the content of that care and this is then used to inform local guidelines regarding the nature of that provision. This means that women across the UK will have different experiences depending on the local model of care.

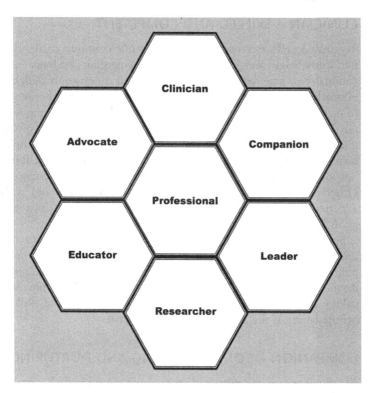

Figure 7.1 The midwife's role: patchwork model

Midwives are the lead professionals for women postnatally and have the role of coordinating the care the woman needs. This responsibility may be shared between herself, the health visitor and infant-feeding support workers; with further input from the general practitioner and obstetrician if there are or have been any medical or obstetric complications. Continuity of midwifery care should continue in the postnatal period so that the woman benefits from not having to repeat her story to midwives she does not know (Sandall et al. 2016). Providing continuity of care is also very rewarding for the midwife and can enhance job satisfaction (Fenwick et al. 2018).

CLINICIAN – SKILLED AND COMPETENT

To provide effective care the midwife must continue to develop her knowledge and skills in light of emerging evidence and national best practice guidelines. Her clinical observation skills are invaluable in the postnatal period; the midwife uses all of her senses to pick up on any cues that the woman is well and recovering well physically and adjusting emotionally to her new role. Some of the midwives' skills are formal and routinely applied; for example, taking measurements of the woman's blood pressure, asking about her lochia and ensuring her breasts are free from signs of mastitis. Other clinical skills are subtler and develop over time and with experience, such as noticing the woman's demeanour, how she holds her baby or sits uncomfortably on her perineal wound.

Some postnatal skills require considerable manual dexterity and supervised practice before they are accomplished; for example, perineal suturing. This important surgical technique requires a detailed knowledge of the anatomy of the pelvic floor, pharmacology of anaesthetising the perineal muscle and skin and skill in manipulation of the needle and suture material.

COMPANION – COMMUNICATING AND NURTURING

As a familiar face and respected professional the midwife has got to know the woman during her pregnancy and understands her social and obstetric circumstances. The midwife may also have had the joy and benefit of being with her during the birth. This relationship now comes into its own at the time when the woman is coming to terms with the birth and realising the impact of caring for her baby. The midwife will use her listening and affirming skills to subtly promote confidence and attunement between the mother and her infant. There are key pieces of information that the midwife must get across to the new parents so that they can make informed decisions about their care. For example, if a woman has chosen to breastfeed, and then through fatigue, external pressure or concern, tells the midwife she wants to give the baby a formula feed, the midwife will need to ensure that the woman understands the consequences. It is difficult sometimes to provide information that is easy to understand in the heat of the moment, and always better to have been able to do this before a crisis occurs. However, the midwife needs to not only give correct information, but in a way that is easy to digest and does not feel judgemental. At the end of the day, the woman can make her own choices, but she should not have regrets that she did not know the consequences of her decision.

ADVOCATE – PROTECTING AND ENABLING

There are times when the midwife needs to take a step forward to act in the best interest of the woman and her baby. In most circumstances, the midwife is facilitating and enabling the new mother to become familiar with her baby's cues and understand its needs. She has sown the seeds during the pregnancy, encouraging the woman to speak to and stroke her baby as it develops and grows. The midwife has encouraged her to respond to its kicks and get to know its patterns of rest and wakefulness. These are all essential skills that the mother will need to continue to care for her baby once it makes its presence in the outside world. The midwife can also support the woman's partner to engage and learn how to respond to the baby's cues and needs. Such supporting comments such as, 'Look at how Phoebe is listening to your voice. She recognises you, look how intently she is looking at you and getting to know your face.' It may seem obvious, but in the blur of emotion and fatigue, sometimes key moments need to be brought to the fore and midwives are so well placed to do this.

EDUCATOR – FACILITATING LEARNING

We all learn differently and in different ways depending on the circumstances. It is suggested (UNICEF 2016) that women who have had a baby are in left brain mode, which means that they find it difficult to take in abstract concepts and need to feel and experience things to understand and absorb them. Indeed, there is increasing evidence that the maternal brain changes throughout the postpartum period and she becomes more responsive to cues from her infant, increasingly empathetic and attuned to the emotional state of the baby (Barba-Müller et al. 2019).

One of the most important ways that the midwife can facilitate learning is through role modelling. Babies provide a fantastic opportunity not only through which to demonstrate skills, but because we often 'talk' to babies as we care for them, we can provide a running commentary about *why* we are doing something too. For example, when a midwife greets the baby in its moses basket at a postnatal home visit, she can say something like, 'Hello, Phoebe, well you are looking a lovely pink colour. Your daddy has made you safe with your feet at the foot of the basket and tucking the cover under your arms. I'll just wash my hands before I look at how your cord is doing.' Opportunities to reiterate safer sleep messages and reducing the risk of infection can be embraced in a simple greeting.

RESEARCHER – CREATOR OF NEW KNOWLEDGE

Midwives are required to provide evidence-based practice wherever possible. Where there is no evidence about how to perform a certain task, she should ask herself, why? When NICE guidelines are developed, the team of experts in the subject area are supported by analysts who are skilled in assessing the quality of the evidence and identifying where there are gaps in the knowledge base. There will be a list of suggested topics requiring further research, some of which ultimately find their way into commissioned calls for investigators to apply for funding from the National Institute for Health Research (NIHR). The current NICE guidance for postnatal care (NICE 2006) identifies areas for research including: what is the cost effectiveness of the Baby Friendly Initiative accreditation programmes compared to another or standard care? Is the severity of postnatal depression among socially isolated women reduced by the provision of peer social support compared with standard care? Does routine monitoring of the weight of all low-risk babies during the first 6–8 weeks after birth reduce the incidence of serious morbidities?

LEADER – CHANGE AGENT

The knowledge base continues to expand and as midwives grow in their capacity to appreciate and evaluate the emerging evidence they then need to be able to influence how care is provided. Leadership can be demonstrated at any level of experience or midwifery role. For example, a student midwife can show leadership by highlighting an area of practice that does not reflect the evidence base and raising this with her mentor. Being prepared to question, and reflect on, practice helps others to take a step back and consider ways that care practices can be shaped or changed for the better. Leadership is shown when a midwife is a role model to her colleagues, always talking with respect to the women she cares for, no matter how many times they have rung the buzzer for support or how near the end of the shift it is when someone needs assistance.

SO, WHAT IS POSTNATAL CARE?

The International Confederation of Midwives (ICM) essential competencies for midwifery practice (ICM 2018) categorises care into:

1 Provide postnatal care for the healthy woman
2 Provide care to healthy newborn infant
3 Promote and support breastfeeding
4 Detect, treat and stabilise postnatal complications in woman and refer as necessary
5 Detect, stabilise and manage health problems in newborn infant and refer if necessary
6 Provide family planning services

These global competencies will be used throughout the chapter to provide a framework to describe the role of the midwife in postnatal care.

PROVIDE POSTNATAL CARE FOR THE HEALTHY WOMAN

REVIEW HISTORY OF PREGNANCY, LABOUR AND BIRTH

When considering how to care for a woman and her baby it is important to know and take account of what has gone before. The midwife reviews the medical and pregnancy history and then considers the birth process and outcome. The impact of events around the birth can have an enduring effect on how a woman feels about her role as a person, mother, partner and daughter. Yet often what a midwife reads in the labour records as an account of the birth is far from how the woman remembers it. It is therefore important that the woman has the opportunity to recount her version of events and for the midwife to be able to interpret or explain why certain things may have happened. For example, it is common for women to have misconceptions about why she needed an emergency caesarean. One woman in the PINK study (Baston 2006) recounted how she had not been part of the decision to have a caesarean, but on reflection was glad not to have that responsibility:

> I just went along with it. I just, you know, I didn't know whether I could say yes or no [...] I didn't know I could have said no. But then you know, if something had happened, I would have thought, 'well, I said no, and look what happened' (174).

NICE (2006) guidance recommends that women have the opportunity to talk about the birth and ask questions. This should happen soon in the postnatal period so that women and their partners are not left confused or troubled by something that has a simple explanation. For some women who do not get this opportunity, questions remain unanswered for years and can be detrimental to how they feel about having another baby. Many maternity units have a specialist midwifery service for women to talk to a senior midwife about their birth experience and this may be many years after the event (see Chapter 8).

CONDUCT A FOCUSED PHYSICAL EXAM

The midwife is skilled in undertaking a top-to-toe examination of the mother in the postnatal period to ensure that return to pre-pregnancy health is on course. However, this is not a routine, one-size-fits-all approach – it should be personalised to the emotional and physical needs of the mother. So, for example, if a woman has a straightforward vaginal birth, then it would be expected that the midwife observes the woman's perineum and if there is not wound or cause for concern, subsequent evaluation can be by talking to the woman about how her perineum feels. If, however, the woman has a bruised and swollen perineal suture site, it would be expected that the midwife continues to observe it until she is satisfied that it is healing well.

As with all aspects of postnatal recovery, the woman should know what to expect, what is normal and when to seek medical advice, and it is the midwife's role to ensure she has this information. For example, the woman should be informed to contact a health professional if: she has pain or difficulty passing urine; offensive smelling lochia; abdominal pain; passing clots; excessive blood loss; chest pain; shortness of breath or pain in her calves; headaches or visual disturbances; fever or shivering.

In the UK, women have their postnatal care provided on the NHS. This usually means that they have a visit from their community midwife the day after they go home, day five for the neonatal blood spot screening test and day 10–11 when their care is transferred to the health visitor.

ASSESS MOOD AND FEELINGS ABOUT MOTHERHOOD AND DEMANDS OF INFANT CARE

ADAPTING TO PARENTHOOD

Whilst having a new baby in the family is usually an overwhelmingly joyous and magical time this is not the case for everyone. Becoming a parent brings with it a huge change in individuals' perception of self. On top of that are the increased demands on time, lack of sleep, unpredictability of events and sometimes disorder. If this is not enough to contend with, the postpartum period can also bring emotional and mental ill health. Then, for women with a pre-existing mental health challenge, such as anxiety, this time of adjustment can be very precarious.

The midwife's role is to help prepare parents for the road ahead, to have realistic expectation of the journey and give them information to increase their knowledge and skills. The midwife must also be on the lookout for changes in the woman's mood and encourage the partner to do the same. Serious mental health conditions can develop insidiously or rapidly and require a skilled and prompt response to facilitate effective treatment and care. It can be a matter of life and death; in England death by suicide remains the leading cause of direct deaths in the year after the end of pregnancy, with a mortality rate of 2.8 per 100,000 maternities (Knight et al. 2018).

For some women, developing a relationship with their baby takes time. One woman in the PINK study described how she did not instantly form an emotional or physical bond with her baby, but when it did eventually develop it was strong, 'we're together like Velcro now (laughter)' (130).

HOME OR HOSPITAL?

The environment that women recover in can have an impact on their well-being and recovery. If a woman and her baby are well after the birth, the best place for her to be to continue her parenting journey is her own home. Of course, that is a huge generalisation; what about the mother who has no social support or who feels that she needs to stay in while she becomes more confident with breastfeeding? The reality is that hospital stays cost money and the emphasis for maternity services to continue to provide a cost-effective service means that most women who are well, despite their individual circumstances, will be encouraged to go home as soon as possible. When a woman is at home, she is more likely to be able to dictate when she eats, sleeps, bathes and dresses, without the pressure of the maternity unit culture that imposes certain timetables to everyday events.

Women in hospital may be disturbed by the routine imposed by changes of shift, handover of staff, drug and doctors rounds and visiting hours. It may not be possible to give women a choice regarding the type of postnatal environment they might prefer. The pressure on postnatal beds and the complexity of the women who needs to be cared for often means that priority is given to women who have a baby on the neonatal unit or who have particular clinical or social needs.

Having your own room in the postnatal period might seem like the luxury option. However, not all women relish this option and many women in the PINK study remembered the loneliness they felt being in a single room. For some women, however, having the privacy of a single room provides sanctuary from the hustle and bustle of the open ward:

It meant, erm, I didn't have to share a room with all these other women and crying babies; it was great (laughs). I had a television and

I, I liked having my own, a single room, because you could just, erm, do what you wanted, and you didn't have to worry about somebody watching you (120).

VISITORS

Everyone wants to be the first to see the new baby, particularly new grandparents who have a dual need to visit – to make sure their own child has survived the journey intact as well as to see which side of the family the new arrival resembles most. Visitors, whether at home or in hospital, can be a mixed blessing; someone to offload and recount their experience to, or someone who needs entertaining and nurturing too. The proliferation of social media and instant sharing of photos, videos and commentary, in theory could make the need to have physically close proximity to the new arrival less pressing, but there is nothing like seeing, holding and smelling a baby that could replace our fascination with them and the stories that surround their birth.

Visiting hours vary between maternity units, most having open access to partners with many having overnight facilities. Enabling other family members and remote nearest and dearest to visit is a contentious issue: when are the new parents to get time to get to know their baby? How is the mother to gain confidence breastfeeding? When can she get some rest? It is not unusual to see maternity wards with many chairs around the bed apparently hemming the woman in, elevated on her pedestal of new mother, while she aches to hold her baby that is being passed around the doting visitors.

PROVIDE PAIN CONTROL STRATEGIES IF NEEDED FOR UTERINE CONTRACTIONS AND PERINEAL TRAUMA

Many women experience pain after childbirth; for example, 'after pains' associated with uterine involution are usually more pronounced in second and subsequent births. Adequate pain relief is essential if the woman is going to be able to focus on feeding and caring for her baby rather than being distracted by pain. The midwife can ensure the appropriate analgesia is prescribed, considering if the woman is breastfeeding and any other medication the woman may be taking.

PROVIDE INFORMATION ABOUT SELF-CARE THAT ENABLES MOTHER TO MEET NEEDS OF NEWBORN

As the woman's advocate, the midwife should try and ensure that the woman has appropriate support so that she can recover in peace. In reality this may be difficult to achieve, especially if the woman has other children to care for or other commitments at home. But encouraging her to accept help where offered and to understand the importance of eating well and taking plenty of fluids can help the woman to cope better with the additional challenges of having a new baby to care for too.

Women also need information about safe exercise after childbirth as physical activity can help women to return to their pre-pregnancy weight, improve muscle tone and improve mood (PHE 2019a).

PROVIDE INFORMATION ABOUT POSTNATAL FAMILY PLANNING METHODS

Mentioning contraception to a newly birthed mother usually elicits such responses as 'never again' or 'he can do his bit now', meaning that the partner is considering vasectomy. Of course, wounds heal quickly, the bleeding stops and sexual intercourse resumes. Women need to know that they can get pregnant before they have another menstrual period, so they can be prepared to choose a contraceptive that suits their needs. Midwives therefore need to keep up to date with the many options available to women and which suit certain circumstances; for example, when women are breastfeeding. The provision of sexual health services varies, so the midwife also needs to be aware of the local options for the women she cares for.

PROVIDE CARE FOR THE HEALTHY NEWBORN INFANT

DISTINGUISH NORMAL VARIATION IN NEWBORN APPEARANCE AND BEHAVIOUR

The normal attitude of a newborn baby is one of flexion and good tone; a well newborn baby is not floppy like a doll. Its skin should be pink and well perfused. Although some babies do develop physiological jaundice as the body breaks down the red blood cells no longer needed to extract oxygen from its mother's circulation, there should be no sign of jaundice in the first 24 hours. The baby is observed for facial and other anomalies, considering the features of its parents. Any concerns or unusual features should be escalated to a neonatologist. For example, a baby with Down's syndrome has features including: poor muscle tone; a short neck and excess skin at the back of the neck; single palmer crease and upward slanting eyes. The midwife may therefore be the first professional to suspect an abnormality and ask for a senior clinical review. The midwife would need to inform the parents of her findings and the reason for referral in a sensitive yet open and honest manner (Baston & Durward 2017).

EXAMINE INFANT AT FREQUENT INTERVALS TO MONITOR GROWTH AND DEVELOPMENTAL BEHAVIOUR

In addition to the top-to-toe examination carried out by the midwife soon after the birth, a further, more detailed clinical examination, 'Newborn and Infant Physical Examination' (NIPE), is undertaken in the first 72 hours of life. This is performed by a person, usually a midwife, who has undertaken additional education and training. The NIPE includes auscultation of the heart, and examination of the hips, eyes and genitalia (PHE 2019b).

ADMINISTER IMMUNISATIONS; CARRY OUT SCREENING TESTS AS INDICATED

The immunisation programme for neonates will be different depending on where the midwife is working. In the UK, midwives only give BCG vaccinations to babies and only to those who are born in areas of the UK where the rates of TB are high or have a parent or grandparent who was born in a country where there's a high rate of TB. Other vaccinations are given by the practice nurse in primary care, under the advice and guidance of the health visitor.

As previously described, NIPE-trained midwives carry out the first full clinical examination, screening for abnormalities. The community midwife (or hospital midwife if the family are still under maternity unit care) will undertake the heel prick blood test that is performed when the baby is five days old, to screen for serious health conditions. This is learned by student midwives under close supervision by their mentor and requires being able to describe the tests to the parents, complete the form accurately, hold the baby safely to secure the required blood samples and dispose of the equipment appropriately.

PROVIDE INFORMATION TO PARENTS ABOUT A SAFE ENVIRONMENT FOR INFANT CARE

Midwives are the source of a wide range of information for parents to support them to provide a safe environment for their baby to thrive. Of particular concern is that the baby has a safe sleeping environment; one that is smoke-free and not too warm. The details about safer sleeping have changed over the years so it is particularly important that new parents are encouraged to share the details with their own parents and others who may have brought their children up with different guidance. This needs to be sensitively conveyed, because parents always want to do the best for their children and we work with what is known at the time.

We now know that the safest position for a baby to sleep is in a clutter-free cot, with a firm washable mattress, in the same room as its parents. The room should be between 16–20 degrees centigrade, and baby should be placed on its back with its feet at the foot of the cot to prevent it wriggling under the covers. Sofas are particularly dangerous sleeping environments for babies as they can become trapped between its back and the cushions (Lullaby Trust 2019). The reality is that many parents bring their baby into bed with them, especially to breastfeed. Babies like and need to be close to their parents, who need information about keeping their baby safe rather than being made to feel guilty.

Care of the umbilical cord is often a source of concern for new parents. The cord stump, clamped and cut at the birth, is a potential site of infection. Current practice in resource-rich countries is to keep the cord clean and dry and leave it to separate without the use of topical agents (NICE 2006). However, in resource-poor settings, antiseptic agents may be applied to reduce the risk of infection (WHO 2014). The midwife will demonstrate to parents how to clean the cord area with water and to observe the surrounding skin for infection. The following section will focus on infant feeding and the importance of keeping the baby close.

PROMOTE AND SUPPORT BREASTFEEDING

PROMOTE EARLY AND EXCLUSIVE BREASTFEEDING WHILE RESPECTING A WOMAN'S DECISION

The World Health Organization and UNICEF (WHO 2018) recommend that women should breastfeed within an hour of birth and exclusively for six months. However, this goal is far from being achieved; for example, in the UK only 1 per cent of infants are fed in this way. Midwives have been chastised for an overzealous approach to encouraging breastfeeding (RCM 2018); conversations with women need to take account of their wishes, establishing what they already know about breastfeeding and to ensure that they are making informed decisions. There is a fine line between ensuring that women have enough information to make an informed decision and not invoking feelings of guilt or regret in women who choose not to or find it difficult.

While midwives can be vocal in their role as breastfeeding advocates, sometimes the support has not always been personalised or kind. One woman in the PINK study described how the staff expected her to be an expert despite the very different circumstances surrounding each of her births:

> So, whilst they were supportive, they were, and caring, I always felt at the back of the mind, my mind that they were thinking, 'well, you should know this because you've had a baby already,' Erm, so they weren't quite as supportive. I think every pregnancy's different, and every birth is different, and it's got to be treated like that, rather than, 'well, you should know it anyway' (127).

Another woman spoke of her determination to succeed and how she made good use of her time in hospital to get the support she needed:

> I was absolutely determined to do it. [...] I remember buzzing for a midwife to come and see that she was latched properly, and was I doing it right [...] they were very very patient, very very good. They told

me that I'd have to persevere, that it may feel unnatural, erm, and that it might not be easy [...] I was determined anyway, so I did (127).

PROVIDE INFORMATION ABOUT FREQUENCY AND DURATION OF FEEDINGS, AND WEIGHT GAIN

Women need to understand the principle of responsive feeding, whereby they are encouraged to feed their baby following both its cues and their desire to nurture (UNICEF 2016). This means that breastfeeding can take place anytime and anywhere, if the baby is hungry, tired, stressed or just wants a cuddle. In fact, there does not need to be any reason; a breastfed baby cannot be over fed. The midwife will show mothers how to recognise when their baby is showing signs of being ready for a feed: pushing its tongue out, moving its head from side to side, sucking fists, rooting and wriggling. It is ideal to feed a baby when it is showing these signs rather than when it is crying and distressed.

If the baby is introduced to formula milk, then there are potential hazards which the family should be aware of. The establishment of a good milk supply is dependent on the baby regularly being breastfed, to stimulate the release of prolactin and the production of milk. If formula milk is introduced the stimulation to produce milk is reduced and the milk supply will begin to dwindle. As milk production is built on a feedback mechanism, if the breasts remain full of milk, because the baby has bottle fed rather than going to the breast, then messages are sent back to the brain to reduce milk production. Introducing formula milk to breastfed babies can also trigger allergic sensitisation in susceptible infants.

Weight gain is an emotive issue and whilst it is expected that infants lose weight before they start to gain it, women are very vulnerable to seeing that their breastfeeding efforts do not result in weight gain in the first few days. It is at this time that they do not feel that they have any milk and are susceptible to undermining comments from friends and relatives, such as, 'Why don't you just give him a bottle?' However, if the woman and her partner have been prepared to expect such weight loss, and know that the baby's stomach is small and can only accommodate small amounts at a time at first, she will understand that, in due course, her milk will come in and the baby will start to gain weight.

PROVIDE SUPPORT AND INFORMATION ABOUT BREASTFEEDING FOR A MINIMUM OF SIX MONTHS

During the first six months babies need no other source of sustenance than breastmilk. Some women decide to curtail breastfeeding their baby because they need or want to return to work. However, ideally ongoing breastfeeding support could be given where employers provide facilities for women to express and store their breastmilk at work. Midwives can provide information about how to do this safely and inform the mother of the ongoing benefits of continued feeding both for her and her baby.

IDENTIFY AND MANAGE BREASTFEEDING PROBLEMS

If women are shown how to recognise effective latching and feeding, then they are less likely to get engorged breasts or suffer from mastitis because the milk is flowing well. Midwives can show women who do experience blocked ducts how to massage the breast, try alternative positions so the baby drains the breast effectively and hand express milk if they become engorged. Helping women understand why problems occur can facilitate looking for the solution. For example, painful feeding is usually solved by ensuring the baby is latched on effectively, which also helps the baby draw the milk easily and supports further milk production.

PROVIDE INFORMATION TO WOMEN BREASTFEEDING MULTIPLE NEWBORNS

Women who birth twins or more can still breastfeed effectively, although they will need determination and support to do so. They will benefit from specialist input and peer support from women who have experienced tandem feeding and discussing other issues associated with multiple birth, such a sleeping arrangements and what support is available from health and other agencies, such as the Twins Trust (see Resources).

REFER WOMEN TO BREASTFEEDING SUPPORT AS INDICATED

If women are aware of the types of support that are available, access to it can enable them to continue feeding in the face of any challenges they encounter. Support takes many forms; however, it is more effective if it is face to face, scheduled and tailored to the needs of the community in which it is offered (McFadden et al. 2017). In the UK, there are a range of community support services and voluntary agencies available to women who encounter feeding problems when they are no longer receiving midwifery care, including breastfeeding cafes, helplines and websites (NHS 2019a).

DETECT, TREAT AND STABILISE POSTNATAL COMPLICATIONS IN WOMAN AND REFER AS NECESSARY

PROVIDE INFORMATION TO WOMAN AND FAMILY ABOUT POTENTIAL COMPLICATIONS AND WHEN TO SEEK HELP

Building on the information that the woman has already received during pregnancy, the midwife continues to be a source of key information about making a good postnatal recovery. Women need to be able to recognise when their health is deteriorating so that they can seek prompt medical advice (NICE 2006). They also need to know how to recognise ill health in their baby. In the UK, women receive a Personal Child Health Record (PCHR) or 'red book' which details many of the warning signs, so that they can refer to it if they have any concerns (NHS 2019b).

ASSESS WOMAN DURING POSTNATAL PERIOD TO DETECT SIGNS AND SYMPTOMS OF COMPLICATIONS

The midwife assesses the woman's physical and emotional well-being at every postnatal contact to ensure that she is returning to pre-pregnancy health and adapting well to motherhood. With her comprehensive knowledge of the physiology of the puerperium, the midwife can identify when recovery is deviating from normal. For example, if the woman reports that her lochia has become more profuse and offensive smelling, the midwife will suspect uterine infection and investigate this further, asking questions about pain, taking her temperature and pulse and palpating her uterus. Postnatal complications can develop quickly and the midwife needs to take swift and appropriate action to prevent the development of life-threatening conditions such as sepsis.

Where there has been continuity of care from the antenatal to the postnatal period, the midwife is the key professional who can monitor changes in a woman's emotional well-being. However, she is not with the woman 24/7 so it is important that her partner and/or other family members are also alerted to key red flag signs that her mental health is deteriorating, including estrangement from her baby, persistent expressions of incompetence as a mother and self-harm (Knight et al. 2018). Women who express suicidal thoughts require an urgent response, not a next-day appointment (Cantwell et al. 2018).

Psychotic illness, although rare (approximately 1–2 per 1,000 women), can develop quickly, even in women with no previous history. Symptoms of postpartum psychosis include: mania, loss of inhibitions, delusions, restlessness and confusion, and is a medical emergency (Baston & Hall 2019).

DEBRIEFING

One aspect of care that has been heralded as a valuable component of postnatal care is 'debriefing' (NICE 2006). There is some confusion regarding the use of this term, which has traditionally been used to describe a structured intervention aimed at preventing psychological morbidity following a traumatic event (Dyregrov 1989). However, the term has also been used to refer to services developed by midwives to help women who have unanswered questions following childbirth (see Chapter 8). One woman in the PINK study expressed her concern that women with difficult births are not routinely offered support:

> I think that everybody's birth experiences are so different and personal to each individual. I'm not happy about either of my births. I felt both were awful and I still feel cheated because I didn't enjoy bringing my children into the world [...] I do feel that more should be done for women who have difficult births as it does stay with you forever (87).

EDINBURGH POSTNATAL DEPRESSION SCALE (EPDS)

In clinical practice this ten-item questionnaire (Cox et al. 1987) is used as a screening tool by health visitors postnatally to identify women at high risk of postnatal depression (those who score over 12), so that they can receive additional professional input. The EPDS is also a measure employed in many research studies; however, Green (2005) urges caution in the way that it is used because to dichotomise women into two groups, based on this cut-off, is to suggest that a woman with a score of 13 is equivalent to someone with a score of 20. She therefore argues that the EPDS should be used as a continuous measure during analysis. Further, as EPDS is a tool that is familiar to women who have had a baby, they may have become adept at providing appropriate rather than honest answers.

PROVIDE FIRST-LINE MEASURES TO TREAT OR STABILISE IDENTIFIED CONDITIONS

The midwife's role is unique in that she not only has a social role as advocate and companion to women, but she also has a front-line clinical role. For example, the midwife needs to be skilled in adult and neonatal resuscitation, know how to deal with emergencies such as cord prolapse or postpartum haemorrhage and manage unexpected breech or premature births. Her swift and appropriate actions save lives and prevent serious maternal and neonatal morbidity.

ARRANGE REFERRAL AND/OR TRANSFER AS NEEDED

The midwife is a practitioner in her own right and is the expert in caring for women experiencing straightforward pregnancies and births. However, she is also part of a wider multidisciplinary team and is obliged to refer to other specialists if she detects a problem or the mother's and/or infant's condition deteriorates. Midwives continue to provide care for women who have been referred, ensuring they continue to receive information about parenting and infant feeding, to continue their transition to parenthood despite any medical or obstetric complications.

The role of the midwife is usually associated with new life and happy times. Sadly, this is not always the case. Fetal or neonatal loss can occur at any time along the pregnancy and postnatal pathway, and the midwife will play a role in supporting and caring for the affected families. She will continue to care for the woman to ensure a return to physical health, and work in collaboration with bereavement services to provide pastoral care. Creating memories is an important aspect of this work, and women and families need to have the opportunity to get to know their baby, perhaps bath and dress the baby, take photographs and foot prints, as a means of acknowledging the important place their child will continue to have in their lives. There are a range of charities, such as the Stillbirth and Neonatal Deaths Society (SANDS) and 4Louis, that can provide peer support for parents as they try and come to terms with their loss.

Midwives also need support and someone they can turn to when a baby dies. She may be asking herself if there was something she missed or could have done differently and this period of reflection is important so that any lessons can be learned to prevent such tragedies happening in the future. Many maternity units have a system in place for reviewing each stillbirth or neonatal death, using a range of criteria to look for patterns and causative factors. Usually there is either an obvious congenital abnormality or an event, such as a placental abruption, which could not have been avoided or predicted.

There are a range of factors associated with infant mortality and hence key work streams to ensure that there are systems in place to mitigate them. One example is the 'Saving Babies' Lives' care bundle (NHS England 2019), which provides a set of standards that maternity units are required to achieve. It includes ensuring best practice around: monitoring the fetal heart in labour; responding appropriately to reports of reduced fetal movement; helping women to quit smoking in pregnancy; reducing preterm birth; and preventing and monitoring babies at risk of fetal growth restriction.

DETECT, STABILISE AND MANAGE HEALTH PROBLEMS IN NEWBORN INFANT

During the routine examinations made by the midwife following birth and subsequent postnatal period, the midwife will recognise when there are characteristics or behaviours in the infant that give her cause for concern. Caring for healthy newborns over time, the midwife becomes skilled in detecting when a baby is not well. There will be situations where the midwife is anticipating and observing for signs and symptoms of ill health; for example, when a mother is a known drug user or if the baby is suspected of having an infection. There will also be times when a healthy term baby develops jaundice, for example, or does not thrive and gain weight. The midwife, in such circumstances, can undertake investigations, such as checking the baby's bilirubin levels or undertaking a feeding assessment following excessive weight loss. If her suspicions are confirmed she must then refer to a specialist, such as a neonatal nurse practitioner or neonatologist for further investigation and potential treatment.

PROVIDE FAMILY PLANNING SERVICES

The midwife not only advises on the most appropriate family planning methods for women but also needs to be able to advise how to use them, especially if a new method is being tried. For example, for women using the traditional Progesterone Only Pill (POP), which is safe during breastfeeding, she needs to know that she should take it within the same three-hour window in order for it to be effective. The desogesterol pill must be taken within a 12-hour window (NHS 2019c).

Family spacing is particularly important for women in countries where unintended pregnancy can not only impact on their physical health, but on their future aspirations and economic prospects. Being able to care for and feed large numbers of children can be a serious challenge. If women are becoming pregnant within a year of giving birth, their risk of morbidity and mortality is significant increased (WHO 2013). Globally, Post Partum Family Planning (PPFP) is therefore seen as a life-saving intervention (WHO 2012) and midwives have an important role in supporting women choose and access methods that suit them.

CONCLUSION

Midwives have an important role in the immediate hours and days after the new baby's arrival. Whilst postnatal care may appear to be less acute and complex compared to the drama of birth, the midwife can offer vital emotional and educational support to new parents through role modelling and sensitive companionship. She also has an important role in monitoring physical and psychological well-being, anticipating and preventing potential complications and enabling new parents to enjoy getting to know and nurture their new baby.

RESOURCES

4Louis, https://4louis.co.uk/. Charity supporting families through miscarriage, stillbirth and child loss.

BASIS – baby sleep info course, www.basisonline.org.uk. A resource for parents and professionals about infant sleeping and safety.

Baston H, and Hall J (2017). *Midwifery essentials, volume 4 – postnatal care.* 2nd ed. London: Elsevier. This pocket textbook for midwives covers a range of postnatal issues including care of the baby, care after caesarean birth, emotional well-being and infant feeding.

Brodrick A, and Williamson E (2020). *Listening to women after childbirth.* London: Routledge.

UNICEF Baby Friendly Initiative (2019), www.unicef.org.uk/babyfriendly/. This website hosts a range of resources that provide evidence and insight into why it is important to support close and loving relationships between the infant and its carers.

UNICEF UK Baby Friendly Initiative (2012), www.babyfriendly.org.uk. The evidence and rationale for the UNICEF UK Baby Friendly Initiative Standards.

Developing NICE guidelines: the manual (NICE 2014, 2018), www.nice.org.uk/process/pmg20/chapter/introduction-and-over view. This resource provides a comprehensive manual for guideline development and a useful glossary of terms and further recommended reading.

Stillbirth and Neonatal Death Charity (Sands), www.sands.org.uk. A charity providing support for parents following baby loss, and supporting research to improve care and reduce the numbers of babies who die.

Twins Trust (formerly Twins and Multiple Birth association (TAMBA)), https://twinstrust.org/. Support network and practical information for parents of twins and multiples.

REFERENCES

Barba-Müller E, Craddock S, Carmona S, and Hoekzema E (2019). Brain plasticity in pregnancy and the postpartum period: links to maternal caregiving and mental health. *Archives of Women's Mental Health* 22(2):289–299.

Baston H (2006). Women's experience of emergency caesarean birth. PhD thesis. University of York, http://etheses.whiterose.ac.uk/14082/.

Baston H, and Durward H (2017). *Examination of the newborn: a practical guide.* 3rd ed. London: Routledge.

Baston H, and Hall J (2019). *Midwifery essentials: emergency maternity care.* Volume 6. London: Elsevier.

Cantwell R, Youd E, and Knight M (2018). Messages for mental health. In *Saving lives, improving mothers' care – lessons learned to inform maternity care from the UK and Ireland confidential enquiries into maternal deaths and morbidity 2014–2016* (ed. Knight M, Bunch K, Tuffnell D, Jayakody H, et al. on behalf of MBRRACE-UK). Oxford: National Perinatal Epidemiology Unit, University of Oxford, www.npeu.ox.ac.uk/downloads/files/mbrrace-uk/reports/MBRRACE-UK%20Maternal%20Report%202018%20-%20Web%20Version.pdf.

Cox J, Holden J, and Sagovsky R (1987). Detection of postnatal depression. Development of the 10-item Edinburgh Postnatal Depression Scale. *The Br J Psychiatry* 150:782–786.

Dyregrov A (1989). Caring for helpers in disaster situations: psychological debriefing. *Disaster Management* 2(1):25–30.

Fenwick J, Sidebotham M, Gamble J, *et al.* (2018). The emotional and professional wellbeing of Australian midwives: a comparison between those providing continuity of midwifery care and those not providing continuity. *Women and Birth* 31(1):38–43.

Green J (2005). What is the EPDS measuring and how should we use it in research? In *Screening for perinatal depression* (ed. Henshaw C and Elliott S). London: Jessica Kingsley Publishers, 141–147.

ICM (2018). Essential competencies for midwifery practice, www.internationalmidwives.org/assets/files/general-files/2019/03/icm-competencies-en-screens.pdf.

Knight M, Bunch K, Tuffnell D, *et al.* (Eds) on behalf of MBRRACE-UK (2018). *Saving lives, improving mothers' care – lessons learned to inform maternity care from the UK and Ireland confidential enquiries into maternal deaths and morbidity 2014–2016.* Oxford: National Perinatal Epidemiology Unit, University of Oxford, www.npeu.ox.ac.uk/downloads/files/mbrrace-uk/reports/MBRRACE-UK%20Maternal%20Report%202018%20-%20Web%20Version.pdf.

Lullaby Trust (2019). Safer sleep for babies: a guide for parents, www.lullabytrust.org.uk/wp-content/uploads/Safer-sleep-for-babies-a-guide-for-parents-web.pdf.

McFadden A, Gavine A, Renfrew M, *et al.* (2017). Support for healthy breastfeeding mothers with healthy term babies. *Cochrane Database of Systematic Reviews* (2), doi:10.1002/14651858.CD001141.pub5.

NICE (National Institute for Health and Care Excellence) (2006, updated 2015). Postnatal care up to 8 weeks after birth. NICE CG37, www.nice. org.uk/guidance/cg37. Accessed 21 September 2019.

NHS (2019a). Breastfeeding help and support, www.nhs.uk/conditions/pregna ncy-and-baby/breastfeeding-help-support/. Accessed 2 November 2019.

NHS (2019b). The personal child health record (red book), www.nhs.uk/con ditions/pregnancy-and-baby/baby-reviews/#redbook. Accessed 2 November 2019.

NHS (2019c). The progesterone only pill. Your contraception guide, www.nhs. uk/conditions/contraception/the-pill-progestogen-only/. Accessed 2 November 2019.

NHS England (2019). Saving babies' lives. Version two. A care bundle for reducing perinatal mortality, www.england.nhs.uk/wp-content/uploads/ 2019/07/saving-babies-lives-care-bundle-version-two-v5.pdf.

PHE (Public Health England) (2019a). Physical activity for women after childbirth, https://assets.publishing.service.gov.uk/government/uploads/ system/uploads/attachment_data/file/829895/6-physical-activity-for-wom en-after-childbirth-birth-to-12_months.pdf.

PHE (Public Health England) (2019b). Guidance: newborn and infant physical examination (NIPE) screening programme handbook, www.gov.uk/governm ent/publications/newborn-and-infant-physical-examination-programme-hand book/newborn-and-infant-physical-examination-screening-programme-handb ook.

RCM (Royal College of Midwives) (2018). Position statement on infant feeding, www.rcm.org.uk/news-views-and-analysis/news/rcm-publishes-new-position -statement-on-infant-feeding.

Sandall J, Soltani H, Gates S, *et al.* (2016). Midwife-led continuity models versus other models of care for childbearing women. *Cochrane Database of Systematic Reviews* (4), doi:10.1002/14651858.CD004667.pub5.

UNICEF (2016). UNICEF UK baby friendly initiative. Responsive feeding: supporting close and loving relationships, www.unicef.org.uk/babyfriendly/ wp-content/uploads/sites/2/2017/12/Responsive-Feeding-Infosheet-Unicef-UK-Baby-Friendly-Initiative.pdf. Accessed 2 November 2019.

WHO (World Health Organization) (2012). Family planning: a health and development issue, a key intervention for the survival of women and children, https://assets.publishing.service.gov.uk/media/57a08a7340f0b649740005d4/ WHO_RHR_HRP_12.23_eng.pdf. Accessed 2 November 2019.

WHO (World Health Organization) (2013). Programming strategies for postpartum family planning, https://apps.who.int/iris/bitstream/handle/

10665/93680/9789241506496_eng.pdf?sequence=1. Accessed 2 November 2019.

WHO (World Health Organization) (2014). Implementing the World Health Organization revised recommendations on cord care, www.healthy newbornnetwork.org/hnn-content/uploads/Final-for-translation_ CWG-Country-Guidance_Jan-19-2018_EN.pdf.

WHO (World Health Organization) (2018). Infant and young child feeding, www.who.int/en/news-room/fact-sheets/detail/infant-and-young-child-feeding. Accessed 1 November 2019.

8

MIDWIFE AS SPECIALIST

INTRODUCTION

In this final chapter we will now reflect on the various roles that the midwife plays during her working day and how she might take on a specialist role in which one or more of these pieces of patchwork (see Figure 8.1) have dominance. However, even when a midwife adopts a specialist role or title, she will inevitably continue to use all of these elements, as she draws on the knowledge and skills that have developed over her career. As Professor Mary Renfrew writes:

> There are many ways of being a midwife – we can work in practice, management, leadership, policy, education, and research. I have had the privilege of working in all of these roles across my career as a midwife, which now spans over 40 years. I am based in a university, and I work across the UK and also internationally. I have led a programme of research on midwifery and maternity care for many years, and I teach students, mostly at postgraduate level. I am also involved in using evidence to inform and develop health policy.
>
> Mary Renfrew, Professor of Mother and Infant Health, UK

The examples that follow are merely that. There are myriad other roles that midwives adopt and create, that form the bedrock of safe and effective care. Some roles are prominent and highly visible, such as the Chief Midwife, and others less so but equally important, such as the role of the bereavement midwife. The following examples are presented to offer a taster of where a career in

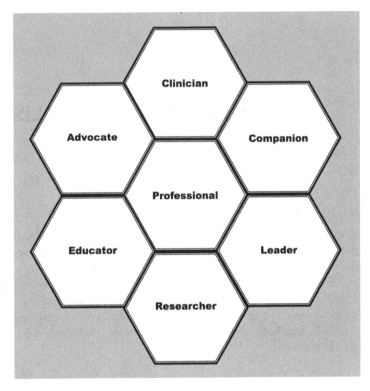

Figure 8.1 The midwife's role: patchwork model

midwifery can lead to. It is a celebration of the legacy and investment of those trailblazers and activists that have enabled midwifery
to be the respected and valued profession it is today.

CLINICAL PRACTICE ROLES

There are a range of opportunities for midwives to specialise in a
particular area of clinical practice, depending on the needs of the
local population and the size, nature and location of the maternity
unit. For example, larger tertiary maternity units are likely to have
more clinical specialist roles, to provide and coordinate care for
women experiencing complicated pregnancies. Units that serve

populations where there are higher rates of consanguinity may invest in specialist midwives to offer culturally sensitive genetic screening opportunities for affected families. In addition to the clinical aspect of providing specialist care, midwives in these roles will also have responsibilities for collating data, meeting national targets and ensuring compliance with national guidance.

PUBLIC HEALTH

All midwives have a public health role, to promote and protect women's well-being during their pregnancy and help them start family life in the best possible state of emotional and physical health. Pregnancy is seen as a 'teachable moment' (RCM 2017) where women are receptive to making positive lifestyle changes, therefore midwives needs to be skilled in making the most of this window of opportunity. They need to be aware of the wider determinants of health, such as poverty, education, employment and economic status to understand the social circumstances of the women they care for (Marshall et al. 2019). The impact of intrauterine life, the birth and early childhood can have a lasting legacy for that child's long-term health and opportunities (Marmot 2010).

There are some midwifery roles that have a specific public health remit and cover a wide range of issues, including the support of flu vaccination programmes, reducing maternal obesity, driving smoking cessation initiatives and working with infant feeding teams. Other public health roles might cover the development of care pathways for women who are subject to a range of vulnerabilities such as substance misuse, domestic violence and the safeguarding requirements that they create. Research commissioned by the RCM found a range of diverse and complex roles fulfilled by midwives working in public health and identified 35 topics (RCM 2017:57).

Many maternity units have invested in the development of a midwife to work specifically with women who have or develop severe mental illness and therefore work across agencies to provide care in liaison with the perinatal mental health teams. Indeed, the 'Long Term Plan' (Department of Health 2019) pledges to increase provision for perinatal mental health services from preconception to up to 24 months, provide care for partners and provide maternity outreach clinics to increase availability and access to evidence-based services.

INFANT FEEDING

The UNICEF Baby Friendly Initiative (BFI) provides a framework for maternity units (and many other facilities where babies are cared for) to achieve high standards of care through the implementations of infant feeding policies, evidence-based staff education and mother-centred support. Through a process of continual audit and assessment of staff skills and women's experiences, units that meet the BFI standards are accredited. However, not all maternity units have gone through this valuable process, and in an attempt to bring our breastfeeding rates in line with the rest of Europe, it has been stipulated in the 'Long Term Plan' (Department of Health 2019) that those units which are not accredited will begin the process by 2020.

At the forefront of leading the process of BFI accreditation and re-accreditation are infant deeding coordinators, who work tirelessly to ensure that the standards are met. These midwives keep the guidelines and infant feeding curricula up to date; coordinate staff and mothers audits; liaise with midwives, peer supporters, clinical support workers and managers to keep the process on track. They are passionate and committed, as Sue clearly demonstrates below:

> Infant feeding decisions ... emotive, inflammatory, sparking passion, deep instinct, fear and guilt. Society is all too ready to state its fickle opinion and damn mothers however they choose to feed their babies. How does a mother navigate these choppy waters without drowning? As an infant feeding lead I am dedicated to equipping mothers with a life jacket, getting in the boat with them and holding their hand through the storm at the beginning of their feeding journey. My role is to help a mother look within herself at the strength, and powerful instincts and intuition that drive her to protect and nurture her baby. To help her tune into her desires, hopes, dreams and concerns for herself and her baby and to be able to express them without fear of judgment or accusation. To be a protection against the barrage of outside influences that aim to knock her confidence and tell her she's not good enough for the job.
>
> What a privilege it is to be part of the start of this journey. To positively support and influence the loving connections made between a

mother and her newborn child and know this is building the best foundations for the whole of their lives.

However, my role goes further still … To empower, equip, enable and encourage others to do the same for all mothers and their families.

Sue Cooper, midwife and infant feeding coordinator, UK

The infant feeding coordinator may be a single voice in a small maternity unit, or lead a team of infant feeding midwives, support workers and volunteers in a larger facility. Either way, their valuable role and drive to improve care for women and families is immeasurable.

SCREENING

Midwives undertake screening observations of the mother and her baby every day as part of their clinical role. These include fetal anomaly screening, infectious diseases, newborn blood spot and sickle cell and thalassaemia screening. In some maternity units, a midwife with a special interest in genetic counselling or infectious disease will have a role in co-ordinating the continuing care of women who screen positive and need to discuss the diagnostic and treatment options.

However, there are some screening functions that require additional expertise and advanced training; for example, examination of the newborn. In the UK, the National Screening Committee (NSC) provide standards and guidance regarding the tests and examinations that should be undertaken on all newborn infants (UK NSC 2019a). The Newborn and Infant Physical Examination (NIPE) clinical check-up is performed on all babies in the UK before they are 72 hours old. The aim of this screening test is to detect and refer babies with congenital abnormalities of the heart, hips, eyes and/or testes as part of a head-to-toe clinical examination (UK NSC 2019b).

This examination was historically undertaken by medical staff; however, following the pioneering work of Michaelides (1997) it is now predominantly performed by midwives or nurses who have undergone an additional programme of education and supervised practice. Midwives are ideally placed to perform this examination; it enables them to offer continuity of care for women and provides a valuable opportunity to pass on public health messages to parents while examining their baby (Baston & Durward 2017). Increasingly newly qualified midwives are exiting their pre-registration midwifery programme having undertaken the theoretical component of a NIPE module. However, they must have also completed the clinical assessment component before they can be deemed competent to perform this role (UK NSC 2019b).

A further role that is being taken on by some clinical midwives is that of midwife ultrasonographer. Ultrasound scanning is an integral part of antenatal care; used for simple pregnancy dating to complex investigations of fetal anatomy. Increasingly midwives are undertaking programmes of further clinical education to develop the skill required to provide a midwifery-led service for women requiring growth and fetal well-being surveillance. This skill requires considerable hand–eye coordination, theoretical knowledge and supervised practice to develop competence. It is another example of an opportunity for midwives to provide important health messages, such as the impact of smoking on fetal growth, whilst undertaking screening for potential growth restriction.

SMOKING CESSATION

Addressing the issue of smoking in pregnancy is everyone's business, so it is important that all members of the maternity care team are familiar with the care pathway. In the UK, smoking in pregnancy guidance is provided by NICE (2010); however, it is high priority in many national policies and care bundles due to its significant contribution to both maternal, fetal and neonatal morbidity and mortality (NHS England 2019).

Smoking cessation services are commissioned in various ways, for example by local authorities (city councils) and clinical commissioning groups, and therefore provided by a range of professionals in different configurations. Where the service is provided by midwives, it is important that the post holders have a good grounding in midwifery care because as women get to know their Smoking Cessation Midwife (SCMW) they will inevitably ask her midwifery related issues, such as questions about fetal movements, how to get free prescriptions or what to do about her indigestion. In order to provide smoking cessation support and advice about pharmacological and non-pharmacological aids, the midwife needs to be trained and assessed at level 2 (NCSCT 2019).

The ideal process for generating a referral to the SCMW is that all women are offered carbon monoxide monitoring having been informed about what it is and why it is offered. If the woman has a raised CO reading (4 parts per million (ppm) or more) the source of that exposure is then explored. The most common source is if she smokes, but if she says she does not then other sources should be considered, such as if she lives with a smoker or has been in a smoker's car. Other sources include faulty gas appliances, a route to work or to the antenatal clinic that is particularly polluted and exposure to wood smoke such as from a wood-burning stove. If the woman is a smoker, it is useful at this stage that the midwife explains what support is available, when and where.

The aim of most smoking cessation services is to help the woman achieve a four-week quit; however, some offer continued support throughout pregnancy. One of the most challenging elements of this role is engaging women. It is therefore important that the booking midwife does a great job in selling the services of the SCMW and making a referral. Women can feel guilty about the fact they are still smoking and will often say that they would like to stop smoking when they are in front of their midwife but then do not respond when the SCMW calls to arrange a meeting. When the SCMW does meet with the woman she will assess her level of nicotine addiction and together plan for the most appropriate way forward for her. Some women want to quit there and then, and others need time to prepare. The SCMW will be a source of support and strength to the woman, whichever path she chooses.

BIRTH AFTERTHOUGHTS

Sometimes a woman has unanswered questions after the birth, perhaps because events rapidly unfolded or she was heavily medicated or unwell. She may wonder why certain decisions were made, who made them or when, but have little recall herself. Such uncertainties can fester for months and years and suddenly re-emerge following an incident or subsequent pregnancy. They may never have gone away. It is at this time that many women reach out to a birth afterthoughts service for a compassionate ear from an experienced midwife who can take her hand through the notes and her help make sense of what happened. This service is provided by a senior midwife, often at consultant level, to ensure that the woman is restored and not harmed by this process, or where further psychological support is needed, appropriate referral is made. Alison Brodrick describes the process and the valuable insights women's stories provide:

> Caring for a woman in labour and supporting her through birth is hugely satisfying, the immediate relief and joy of the woman and her partner as they greet their new baby is unique and magical to all. For many women, however, this immediate postnatal period is not accompanied by 'instant love' and during the days and weeks that follow some women are left feeling empty and hollow. When women attend birth afterthoughts, they often have large gaps in their memory of birth events and often beat themselves up for not doing it the way that they themselves had hoped or that society portrays as best. In addition, it never ceases to amaze me just how harsh women can be on themselves, their narrative often punctuated with feelings of inadequacy, distress and guilt. I have learnt to actively listen with minimal interruptions, allowing women to ventilate their feelings and tell their story, often for the first time.
>
> As I start to unpick the facts and explain what actually happened, women will often say 'but no one explained that ...' or 'wow ... I never knew that, so it wasn't my fault then?' As they start to assimilate this new knowledge alongside their own interpretation of events a new narrative becomes possible. To see the tension and insecurity dissipate is hugely rewarding. But what I enjoy most is helping women to see just how amazing they are, highlighting to them all they have achieved through pregnancy, childbirth and as a new mum, thus giving them permission to feel proud. In addition, listening to women's narratives offers us a unique lens to reflect on our own practice as midwives. It is humbling and sometimes upsetting to hear how our everyday language or clinical actions can be interpreted negatively by women. It is important to listen, important to learn and important to women that we use their narratives to adapt and change our practice.

Alison Brodrick, consultant midwife, UK

BEREAVEMENT

Sadly, stillbirth and neonatal loss accounted for 5.4 per 1,000 total births in the UK in 2017 (Draper et al. 2019). Whilst this rate is coming down, it represents the loss of more than 4,000 lives before, during or up to a month after birth, each year.

Some women will know during pregnancy that their baby is unlikely to survive, either because of a genetic abnormality or because of an antenatal event. In such circumstances, a woman may be offered a termination of pregnancy. The woman would then have her labour induced and she would give birth to a still-born baby. For some parents this may be a sad, yet straightforward decision, and others will agonise over whether this will be the right decision for them. Every situation is unique and experienced differently, indeed some parents will decide to continue with the pregnancy and await events to take their course. Most maternity units have a midwife who is dedicated to caring for women in these circumstances, who knows how to offer culturally sensitive care and provide information about registering the birth and making funeral arrangements.

A national bereavement care pathway has been launched (SANDS 2019) to support best practice and ensure that there is a framework for the provision of personal, sensitive care to parents when their baby dies. Bereavement midwives have an important role in being a source of information for other midwives, ensuring that the principles of best practice are incorporated into continuing professional development opportunities for their colleagues. In some maternity units, the bereavement midwife is also involved in the care of women in subsequent pregnancies. When a woman has had a previous stillbirth, she is likely to be fearful of the future and planning for another baby. If she has access to a midwife who knows her journey and can take her specific circumstances into account, she can approach her next pregnancy with less trepidation (Power et al. 2017).

MANAGEMENT, LEADERSHIP AND POLICY

For a midwifery leader, at whatever level, maintaining credibility is essential. It is important that those who are being led appreciate that their senior colleagues understand what life is like, from their perspective. Some senior leaders use the concept of 'back to the floor' (Jones & Griffiths 2011) to demonstrate that they value and truly grasp what midwives in the clinical areas are doing on a day-to-day basis. Others use alternative means such as 'surgeries' or 'drop-ins' to facilitate staff engagement and maintain their visibility. Midwifery leaders represent the profession; here are a few examples of midwife ambassadors.

HEAD OF MIDWIFERY

The number and range of senior management roles will depend on the size of the maternity unit and how it integrates with the wider NHS Trust it is part of. For example, in maternity units that are part of a small district general hospital, there may be only one or two midwifery matrons to support the Head of Midwifery. Matrons oversee the safe and effective running of the wards and departments they are responsible for, and are themselves supported by senior midwifery sisters in the clinical areas.

In larger units, where the Head of Midwifery is also a Director of Nursing Services and therefore overseeing a range of clinical specialities, there will be a more elaborate supportive structure to ensure that senior leadership reaches all corners of the service. Responsible for the strategic vision of the maternity service, the Head of Midwifery has a highly influential role in steering the future direction and profile of the service, as demonstrated in the following vignette:

> The Head of Midwifery (HOM) is a leadership role which involves enabling a team of midwives and maternity support workers to provide optimal clinical care to meet the needs of women and their families. For this to be effective as the HOM I am required to facilitate a culture which enables women to make their own decisions throughout pregnancy, birth and the postnatal continuum. To support continual improvement, I aim to facilitate a positive environment which promotes individuality, diversity and evidence-based practice. I have a responsibility to ensure that I foster a progressive vision for the service which embodies the clinical choices women consider important; whilst integrating local and national initiatives.

The maintenance of professional standards is of primary concern to me as the HOM to ensure that the midwives are appropriately supported, skilled and regulated to provide best clinical practice. To manage successful professional development, I aim to ensure that the profile of midwifery is represented within the organisation, across partnership organisations and the wider NHS; including the midwifery professional body. There is a finite maternity budget and as the HOM I must ensure that this public money is spent wisely in the strategic development of the service and workforce planning and modernisation. I am therefore highly committed to succession planning for future clinicians, managers, educators and researchers. It is imperative that the maternity service and the midwifery team are developed so that they flourish and move forwards in an ever-evolving clinical environment.

As the HOM I hold a privileged position; I am a guardian and custodian of the service during my time in post. It is therefore essential that I coach a team of midwives who value lifelong learning, ongoing personal and professional development, and who implement contemporaneous evidence-based practice.

Paula Schofield, Head of Midwifery, UK

CONSULTANT MIDWIFE

The role of the consultant nurse and midwife was first heralded in the government strategy document 'Making a Difference' (Department of Health 1999). The vision was to provide a career structure which valued senior clinical staff enabling them to remain in practice for 50 per cent of their time. It was stated that:

Nurse, midwife and health visitor consultants will have responsibilities in four main areas: expert practice; professional leadership and consultancy; education and development; and practice and service development linked to research and evaluation. The weight attributable to each of these areas will vary from post to post depending on the particular needs and service in which they are established (Department of Health 1999:33).

The roles continued to be promoted, and further government strategy, 'Maternity Matters' (Department of Health 2007), promoted increasing innovative roles, investing in the development of new skill sets, including the role of the consultant midwife. It was stated that:

> Consultant midwives provide senior clinical leadership within maternity services and complement the role of the Head of Midwifery. Consultant midwives contribute to effective leadership, training and mentoring, as well as having specific responsibilities such as promoting normal birth or reducing inequalities. Consultant midwives are able to drive services improvement through working with colleagues in health and other agencies to develop effective care pathways or services for specific client groups (Department of Health 2007:43).

Today the majority of consultant midwife roles are in the remit of normal birth, with some focusing on public health. Some consultant midwives maintain clinical contact by running clinics to support women's choice, reducing caesarean sections or birth afterthoughts; others have specific add-on responsibilities such as research or education. Many of the roles now include management and on-call responsibilities to provide further flexibility of support to the management team (Wilson et al. 2018).

PROFESSOR OF MIDWIFERY

Being based in a university and having responsibility for providing academic leadership and teaching excellence is a tall order. There are increasing numbers of midwifery professors although getting to such a position remains challenging and requires considerable personal dedication. To be eligible to apply for such a post requires a significant research profile, often of an international calibre. Academics are required to attract research funding and publish their work in peer-reviewed academic journals. In addition, they must attract PhD students and demonstrate the impact of their work. Professors take many different routes depending on their interests. Professor Mary Renfrew has many interests that have had an extensive reach globally, as her most recent work demonstrates:

> I have had a leading role in two projects in the past year. One has been to write a report with the World Health Organization on how best to strengthen education for midwives across the world. In some

countries, midwifery education is weak, and as a result midwives may not have the knowledge and skills they need to work safely with women and babies. To write the report I worked closely with global organisations and attended workshops with midwives from across the world, listening to their views on how to strengthen midwifery education. We were able to use the ideas we heard, along with evidence from research studies, to develop a global action plan for providing good quality midwifery education. This plan is now being implemented in many countries.

The second project was to develop new standards for the education of midwives in the UK. Called the Future Midwife project, it was set up by the Nursing and Midwifery Council (NMC), the organisation responsible for the regulation of midwifery in the UK – they set the education standards that all midwives must reach to be registered and allowed to practise. Working with a team from the NMC, we travelled across the whole UK to listen to midwives, students, women and families, advocacy groups, obstetricians, professional organisations, and many others. We combined the thoughts and ideas that we heard with the best evidence, to develop a set of education standards that will now be taught across all the UK universities and that we hope will help new midwives to give the best possible care.

My work as a midwife working in research, education, and policy is very different from the work of a midwife in practice, but my main aim is the same – to help to ensure the best care possible for all women and babies.

Mary Renfrew, Professor of Mother and Infant Health, UK

Mary has had an inspirational career and continues to raise the aspirations of midwifery and midwives globally. As one of the co-ordinators of the *Lancet* series (see Chapter 1) she appreciates that there is much work to do to take this work forward, 'we have only just started something here' (Holmes 2014).

CHIEF MIDWIFERY OFFICER

In the UK there has been a long history of a Chief Nursing Officer supporting safety initiatives and progressive workforce development. However, it has taken until 2019 to see the first Chief Midwifery Officer in the appointment of Dame Jacqueline

Dunkley-Bent. Her role is to lead the maternity transformation programme outlined in the maternity strategy 'Better Births' (National Maternity Review 2016), which focuses on providing safe maternity care in services that offer continuity of carer within a personalised model of care. Her role will also go beyond this programme and focus on the development of the midwifery workforce, which will aim to make midwifery a career of choice that can be sustained through the diversity of opportunities it provides. The future is looking bright for midwifery with the ambition that midwives can have both their clinical and academic careers recognised as symbiotic rather than having to take either one path or the other (Health Education England 2018).

GOVERNANCE

The concept of clinical governance was introduced into the health service in England following the publication of the strategy document 'A First Class Service: Quality in the New NHS' (Department of Health 1998). It outlined how the National Institute for Clinical Excellence (now National Institute for Health and Care Excellence) would set clear service standards to avoid variation care and that these standards would be monitored through clinical audit processes. Also, staff would be expected to undertake lifelong learning to be able to implement them effectively. This would provide a framework for continually improving the quality of care. Since then, many systems and processes have been developed across health services to ensure that 'patients get the right care at the right time from the right person and that it happens right first time' (NHS England 2017a:12).

Implementation of clinical governance in maternity care has meant that midwives have taken on new and complementary roles to facilitate the running of safe and effective services. One key element of this is having data about clinical outcomes so that services can monitor how well they are doing, especially in relation to their peers and over time. Midwives involved in this work may therefore collate and analyse outcome data and populate dashboards that show trends in these 'clinical quality improvement metrics' (NHS Digital 2019). They may undertake clinical audits to monitor how a particular NICE guideline is being implemented to identify where improvements need to be made. Governance midwives are often involved in the development of local guidelines, investigating clinical incidents and ensuring that complaints are dealt with in an open and transparent manner in line with principles of 'duty of candour' (CQC 2015).

EDUCATION

Education is part of the midwife's role wherever she works; whether it be working with families in preparation for birth, teaching parents about the principles of safer sleeping techniques or showing a woman how to hand express her breastmilk. Midwives also work with a range of staff who are learning on the job, such as student midwives, maternity support workers and medical students. However, midwives can choose to take up a career focusing on the educational needs of pre- and post-registration midwives.

LECTURER IN MIDWIFERY

Some midwives choose to pursue a university-based career, with the aspiration of contributing to the development of future generations of midwives, as passionately described by Sally in Chapter 4. To be eligible to do this, a midwife would need a master's degree and increasingly, a PhD is also essential. A teaching qualification is also desirable, although most universities have their own in-house programme that its staff can access whilst learning the job. With further experience, such academic midwives can take on additional roles within midwifery education such as programme leader, personal tutor, admission's tutor, disabilities coordinator and so on. Where there is also a Professor of Midwifery in the university department, there will often be opportunities to engage in research and reciprocal arrangements for active researchers to contribute to the midwifery curriculum.

Taking the leap into academia is no easy ride. Lecturers often work long hours, writing lectures, developing modules, marking assignments and supporting students in clinical practice. However, it provides the prospect of accessing broader university activities and collaborating with academics from a range of disciplines, and can therefore be an incredibly rewarding path to take.

CLINICAL EDUCATOR

As we have seen in Chapter 4, qualifying as a midwife is only the beginning of a career that requires midwives to engage in lifelong learning and continuing professional development. To support midwives in clinical areas as they further enhance their skills are a range of clinical educators who devote their time to providing educational sessions and one-to-one tuition and practice supervision. When newly qualified midwives start out in the big world of responsibility as a registrant, clinical midwifery educators can be a valuable lifeline to them. They coordinate their preceptorship programme and help induct staff into the workings of the unit. Depending on the size of the unit, there may be a team of educators, each with a particular remit and area of expertise. For example, one may come from a core labour ward background and support staff to develop suturing or epidural top-up skills, whereas another may lead on the support of midwives new to community midwifery.

Clinical midwifery educators are experienced midwives who maintain their practice competence, integrating theory and practice for newly qualified and newly appointed midwives. They must be clinically credible and so often combine their role with clinical shifts, so they can maintain their skills and also work with preceptees in the ward environment. Their roles complement those of preceptors and the learning environment managers, and they often provide a valuable listening ear, as well as practical guidance following challenging clinical situations. Clinical educators are invaluable when new technical equipment comes into the clinical arena, providing support and guidance as new ways of working are embedded.

PROFESSIONAL

As previously discussed, the Nursing and Midwifery Council (NMC) undertake the regulatory function for setting standards and maintaining the midwives' professional register. Until 2017, the voice of midwifery was represented at the NMC by a Midwifery Committee, influencing policy, midwifery standards and the statutory supervision of midwives (see PMA below). This advisory function has now been overtaken by the Midwifery Panel; although it provides 'high-level' advice, insight and assurance, it has no decision-making powers (NMC 2019).

PROFESSIONAL MIDWIFERY ADVOCATE (PMA)

Since 1902 (Midwives Act 1902) midwives were supported in their professional practice by the role of 'supervisor of midwives' (SOMs). These senior midwives provided 24/7 advice and guidance to a caseload of midwives, ensured they were keeping up to date and were fulfilling their statutory requirements and provided a listening ear as a 'critical friend'. They also supported midwives following a difficult or upsetting birth and were a point of contact for women who needed support exercising their choices for birth. However, in direct conflict with these elements of their role, SOMs were also required to investigate allegations of malpractice, negligence or misconduct. Following a number of critical incidents, the role of the SOM was scrutinised (Kirkup 2015). Whilst the supportive and advocacy roles were heralded as relevant and valuable, the investigatory elements were not judged to be fit for purpose, and in March 2017, the role was removed from statute.

It was recognised that an alternative model for clinical midwifery supervision would be required to support midwives in their role, and following a period of consultation, the A-EQUIP (Advocating and Educating for Quality ImProvement) model was launched (NHS England 2017b). This model comprises three functions: restorative supervision, personal action for quality improvement and education and development. It is an employer-led system of support and as such open for individual maternity services to implements in whatever way best meets the needs of their workforce and the challenges they face.

The role of the Professional Midwifery Advocate (PMA) was launched to facilitate this programme. Midwives who had been previous SOMs could access a short bridging course and further opportunities for new PMAs are now provided by universities. PMAs are not required to be on call or investigate poor practice. The main element of their role is new to midwifery and involves supporting midwives to build resilience through restorative supervision. Sessions can take place in groups or one-to-one and build on a confidential relationship where the midwife is listened to and feels heard. It is a non-directive approach, supporting midwives to find their own solutions through reflection.

Midwives are exposed to a range of external stressors at work, especially when caring for women who experience fetal loss. Restorative supervision provides an opportunity to think about and process events, restoring midwives' capacity to provide compassionate care (Wallbank 2013).

PROFESSIONAL STEWARDSHIP

Midwives at all levels can engage with their professional union and take further training to become workplace representatives and advise members on issues around health and safety at work, offer support following a clinical incident and guidance on the rights and benefits of employees. There are a range of unions that midwives can join, some supporting a range of healthcare workers, such as UNISON, and others that are a branch of the nursing union, such as the Royal College of Nursing (RCN) or midwifery specific such as the Royal College of Midwives (RCM).

The professional profile of midwifery is also championed by the RCM, a midwifery organisation that provides advocacy, medicolegal advice and support and learning resources for its members. It also engages in policy debates and sound bite to represent the midwifery and maternity support worker voice. Midwives can undertake courses to become workplace stewards and advise members on issues around employment law, equality legislation and human resources. There is recognition that supporting midwives in the workplace can in turn enhance the care that women and families receive, as articulated by Gill Walton, Chief Executive Officer (CEO) of the RCM:

> I am proud to be a midwife. This is the best job in the world – in all its guises. The relationship that develops with the pregnant woman and the new mother is the most pivotal part of being a midwife and gives rise to huge opportunities to influence the mother and her health choices; supporting her to do the best for herself and her baby. I remain fascinated by the journey women from all walks of life take as they grow into motherhood. I am equally fascinated in how midwives can facilitate and empower women to become stronger and focussed during pregnancy and birth. They often develop deep profound relationships with women over a very short space of time

which can have a transformative effect. Being a midwife is more than delivering babies!

I feel hugely privileged to support midwives, students and maternity support workers to be the best they can be. I build on my knowledge and experience of listening to our members to ensure there is a midwifery voice at every decision-making table. If we can't get it right at the start of the life course, we miss such an opportunity. Midwives are the intervention that makes a difference to all women in the UK and around the world. My vision is to continue to strengthen our profession for every woman, everywhere, because women and babies deserve a transforming start in life.

Gill Walton, CEO and General Secretary,
Royal College of Midwives, UK

RESEARCH

A midwife can be involved in research at a range of levels. It starts during her pre-registration midwifery programme, when the student midwife is undertaking reviews of the research on a chosen topic and learning how to find and critique the published evidence. When the midwife works clinically, she will become aware of research studies that women are being asked to take part in; such as trying a new method for induction of labour or trying a new technology to evaluate wound healing. Whilst not recruiting to the studies herself, she may be asked to give information about the studies to eligible women.

In large teaching hospitals where there is maternity provision, there is likely to be a research department where research activity is coordinated. Whilst supporting research is every registrant's responsibility (NMC 2018), the running of large research studies is a complex speciality which requires a detailed knowledge of the essential governance requirements involved. There are a range of systems and processes that need to be undertaken and followed before a research study can be undertaken. Each department will have a local research co-ordinator who has responsibility for having an overview of the studies currently in progress and who can be a point of contact for any enquiries and research midwives who cater for the operational management of the studies. The research co-ordinator will be supported by a central team providing further expertise on financial and research governance issues as required.

RESEARCH MIDWIFE

When a research team approaches an NHS Trust to ask if it wants to be involved in a research study, the research co-ordinator will direct the request to someone with the clinical expertise in that area. So, for example, if an academic from a local university wants to run a study to test an intervention for promoting exercise in pregnant women, the research co-ordinator will contact the lead for public health to establish if the protocol would fit in with the way that care is organised. The co-ordinator would also ask the research midwives if the protocol design is feasible to implement in the local context, enabling women to be successfully recruited and consented to the study. Together they would explore if, given their pregnant population and the current care pathways, the research would likely be something the team could take on. They would look at the funding that comes with the study and what other resources could be available to support the work, such as additional administrative support from the wider Trust's Clinical Research Facility (CRF).

Research midwives are usually midwives who have comprehensive clinical experience and who have a strong desire to contribute to the increasing body of knowledge that supports contemporary practice. They may have a wish to undertake their own research at some point and want to undertake this role in order to get some wider experience of the governance and recruitment issues involved in running studies. Whatever their motivation, research midwives are key to studies reaching their recruitment targets as they are often the interface between the research protocol, which is the recipe for the study, and gathering the data, or the key ingredients, to answer the research question. They need to have a high level of attention to detail, because the research protocol must be followed to the letter.

When a study is running, the research midwives will need to upload data to appropriate secure digital databases, identify and inform the Principal Investigator (PI) if there are any incidents that happen to participants and ensure they are achieving their recruitment targets. Ideally, they will also be involved in the preliminary stages of research study design, so they can feed their expertise into the development of the protocol, to ensure it reflects current clinical practice and its aims are achievable. They may be involved in supporting the process of seeking ethical approval for local PIs and also sit on Patient and Public Involvement (PPI) panels. In order to function in this role, take consent to studies and manage accurate data collection, research midwives must undertake and maintain Good Clinical Practice (GCP) training. This comprehensive research governance overview outlines the legal and ethical issues associated with research as well as enabling researchers from a range of disciplines to discuss and share their research experiences.

MIDWIFERY RESEARCHER

To be a researcher requires additional education and training, usually beginning with a research module and dissertation at master's level and then a PhD. It requires all of the skills described in the role of the research midwife, and includes the ability to formulate a research question and operationalise that into a workable protocol. One of the main stumbling blocks for midwives who want to be researchers is funding; education costs money and running research studies also requires securing sufficient funds to cover the costs of researcher and often clinician time, technical hardware and software as well as consumables. Although there are many funding streams available, these are highly competitive and it requires considerable time and determination to formulate a plan and galvanise a robust research team, to put together a bid. However, being awarded funding can be life-changing, and the opportunities that open up are to be relished, as Marlies explains:

> I started as an independent midwife in a community setting immediately after midwifery school. After 10 years I really felt the urge to use my brains in a more challenging way and decided to follow an intensive epidemiology course. One thing led to another and within one year I was approached by our national institute for applied research to work for their department of Prevention and Child Health. It was a big change, from daily practice, working with women and their families to an office job. But it was also an exciting change. It felt as if I could contribute to the improvement and strength of midwifery care from a whole different angle: persuade people to change with facts and not just personal beliefs. Within the job I was really free to design

research projects, while listening to care providers, professional organizations, government and clients to which research was needed. I had to motivate care providers to work with me on research and it felt great to finally share the outcomes with them and try to change care to be better. It was not a boring office job, it was a lot of being out there in the field, listening, improvising and the fun of analysing. Discovering new insights does make you feel like Inspector Morse every so often. It made me travel all over the world and to meet wise and interesting people. And on top of that, I was also rewarded personally by achieving a PhD degree.

At this moment I am very involved in a topic that has stolen my heart: group care as another model of health care, not only prenatal but in all domains where people benefit from (peer) support and a holistic approach aimed at positive health. Research into the effects, determining factors of effects and implementation worldwide, the development for different populations and domains: all of that will keep me a very enthusiastic and privileged researcher for the next decade at least.

Marlies Rijnders, midwife researcher, the Netherlands

CONCLUSION

There are so many different routes that a midwife can take during her midwifery career, each invaluable to the creation of the huge patchwork quilt of safe maternity care. Whether the midwife remains in clinical practice or adopts a new role that takes her away from the woman's side, being a midwife is a privilege. No two women, shifts, babies or colleagues are the same; every day is a joy or a challenge, usually both, but the opportunity to make a difference to someone's future is empowering and uplifting.

RESOURCES

Burgess H, Andrzejowska M, Godwin B, et al. (2018). Birth thoughts clinic in Barnsley: who is attending? *Bjog: An International Journal of Obstetrics and Gynaecology* 125, S2:43.

Maternal Health Alliance (2013). Specialist mental health midwives. What they do and why they matter, https://maternalmenta

lhealth.org.uk/wp-content/uploads/2015/09/SMHM-What-they-do-and-why-they-matter.pdf. Includes standards for care, a case study and example job description.

NHSE and NHS Improvement (2019). Developing allied health professional leaders: a guide for trust boards and clinicians, https://improvement.nhs.uk/resources/developing-allied-health-profes sional-leaders-guide/. This guide provides a framework for those allied health professional who are exploring an academic career.

NHS jobs: midwifery vacancies, www.nhsjobs.com/job_list/Nur sing_and_Midwifery/. This website provides insight into the wide range of midwifery roles available in contemporary midwifery.

NHS screening programmes. E-learning for health, www.e-lfh. org.uk/programmes/nhs-screening-programmes/. This website pro-vides a catalogue of e-learning modules across the range of screening programmes on offer in the UK.

Public Health England (2019). Antenatal and newborn screening animation, https://phescreening.blog.gov.uk/2019/09/18/give-us-your-views-on-the-antenatal-and-newborn-screening-animation/.

Royal College of Obstetricians and Gynaecologists (2014). Each baby counts, www.rcog.org.uk/en/guidelines-research-services/a udit-quality-improvement/each-baby-counts/. Video on human factors and situational awareness. Links to reports of the progress to reduce the number of babies who die by 50 per cent by 2020.

REFERENCES

Baston H, Durward H (2017). *Examination of the newborn: a practical guide*. 3rd ed. London: Routledge.

CQC (Care Quality Commission) (2015). Regulation 20: duty of candour, www.cqc.org.uk/sites/default/files/20150327_duty_of_candour_guidance_final.pdf. Accessed 6 November 2019.

Department of Health (1998). A first class service: quality in the new NHS, https://webarchive.nationalarchives.gov.uk/20110322225724/http://www.dh.gov.uk/en/Publicationsandstatistics/Publications/PublicationsPolicyAndGuidance/DH_4006902. Accessed 6 November 2019.

Department of Health (1999). Making a difference: strengthening the nursing, midwifery and health visiting contribution to health and healthcare, https://webarchive.nationalarchives.gov.uk/20120524072447/http://www.dh.gov.uk/prod_consum_dh/groups/dh_digitalassets/@dh/@en/documents/digitalas set/dh_4074704.pdf.

Department of Health (2007). *Maternity matters: choice, access and continuity of care in a safe service*. London: House of Commons.

Department of Health (2019). The NHS long term plan, www.longtermplan.nhs.uk/wp-content/uploads/2019/08/nhs-long-term-plan-version-1.2.pdf.

Draper E, Gallimore I, Smith L, *et al.* (2019). *MBRRACE-UK perinatal mortality surveillance report, UK perinatal deaths for births from January to December 2017*. Leicester: The Infant Mortality and Morbidity Studies, Department of Health Sciences, University of Leicester.

Health Education England (2018). Clinical academic careers framework: a framework for optimising clinical academic careers across healthcare professions, www.hee.nhs.uk/sites/default/files/documents/2018-02%20CAC%20Framework.pdf. Accessed 20 November 2019.

Holmes D (2014). Mary Renfrew: researcher, reformer, midwife. *The Lancet* 384 (9948):1089, www.thelancet.com/journals/lancet/article/PIIS0140-6736(14)61664-0/fulltext. Accessed 3 November 2019.

Jones K, and Griffiths L (2011). Back to the floor Friday: evaluation of the impact on the patient experience. *Journal of Nursing Management* 19(2):170–176.

Kirkup B (2015). *The report of the Morecambe Bay investigation*. London: The Stationery Office, https://assets.publishing.service.gov.uk/government/uploads/system/uploads/attachment_data/file/408480/47487_MBI_Accessible_v0.1.pdf. Accessed 4 November 2019.

Marmot M (2010). Fair society, healthy lives: the Marmot review, www.instituteofhealthequity.org/resources-reports/fair-society-healthy-lives-the-marmot-review/fair-society-healthy-lives-full-report-pdf.pdf. Accessed 6 November 2019.

Marshall J, Baston H, and Hall J (2019). *Midwifery essentials: public health*. Volume 7. London: Elsevier.

Michaelides S (1997). Newborn examination: whose responsibility? *British Journal of Midwifery* 5(9), doi:10.12968/bjom.1997.5.9.538.

National Maternity Review (2016). Better births: improving outcomes of maternity services in England, www.england.nhs.uk/wp-content/uploads/2016/02/national-maternity-review-report.pdf.

NICE (National Institute for Health and Care Excellence) (2010). Smoking: stopping in pregnancy and after childbirth. Public health guideline [PH26], www.nice.org.uk/guidance/ph26.

NCSCT (National Centre for Smoking Cessation and Training) (2019). Training and assessment programme, www.ncsct.co.uk/publication_training-and-assessment-programme.php. Accessed 5 November 2019.

NHS Digital (2019). Maternity dashboard: clinical quality improvement metrics, https://digital.nhs.uk/data-and-information/data-collections-and-data-sets/data-sets/maternity-services-data-set/maternity-services-dashboard. Accessed 6 November 2019.

NHS England (2017a). Implementing better births. A resource pack for local maternity systems, www.england.nhs.uk/wp-content/uploads/2017/03/nhs-guidance-maternity-services-v1-print.pdf.

NHS England (2017b). A-EQUIP: a model of clinical midwifery supervision, www.england.nhs.uk/wp-content/uploads/2017/04/a-equip-midwifery-supervision-model.pdf. Accessed 4 November 2019.

NHS England (2019). Saving babies' lives. Version two. A care bundle for reducing perinatal mortality, www.england.nhs.uk/wp-content/uploads/2019/07/saving-babies-lives-care-bundle-version-two-v5.pdf.

NMC (Nursing and Midwifery Council) (2018). The Code. Professional standards of practice and behaviour for nurses, midwives and nursing associates, www.nmc.org.uk/globalassets/sitedocuments/nmc-publications/nmc-code.pdf. Accessed 16 September 2019.

NMC (Nursing and Midwifery Council) (2019). NMC midwifery panel terms of reference, www.nmc.org.uk/globalassets/sitedocuments/councilpapersanddocuments/terms-of-reference—midwifery-panel-2018.pdf. Accessed 5 November 2019.

Power A, Rea T, and Fenton S (2017). Life after death: the bereavement midwife's role in later pregnancies. *British Journal of Midwifery* 25(5):329–331.

RCM (Royal College of Midwives) (2017). *Stepping up to public health: A new maternity model for women and families, midwives and maternity support workers.* London: Royal College of Midwives, www.rcm.org.uk/media/3165/stepping-up-to-public-health.pdf. Accessed 6 November 2019.

SANDS (Stillbirth and Neonatal Death Society) (2019). National bereavement care pathway, https://nbcpathway.org.uk. Accessed 4 November 2019.

UK NSC (National Screening Committee) (2019a). UK National Screening Committee, www.gov.uk/government/groups/uk-national-screening-committee-uk-nsc. Accessed 6 November 2019.

UK NSC (National Screening Committee) (2019b). Newborn and infant physical examination (NIPE) screening programme handbook, www.gov.uk/government/publications/newborn-and-infant-physical-examination-programme-handbook/newborn-and-infant-physical-examination-screening-programme-handbook. Accessed 6 November 2019.

Wallbank S (2013). Recognising stressors and using restorative supervision to support a healthier maternity workforce: a retrospective, cross-sectional, questionnaire survey. *Evidence Based Midwifery* 11(1):4–9.

Wilson C, Hall L, and Chilvers R (2018). Where are the consultant midwives? *British Journal of Midwifery* 26(4):254–260. Accessed 30 October 2019.

GLOSSARY

Access   The extent to which people are able to receive the information, services or care they need.

Accoucheur   Person assisting childbirth, usually obstetrician or midwife.

Amniocentesis   A procedure which uses a fine needle to draw off amniotic fluid from around the baby. It is done via the maternal abdomen, under scan observation to protect the baby and to find a pool of liquor. The fetal cells in the fluid are then tested for a range of conditions.

Anti-diuretic hormone (ADH)   A hormone which increases the reabsorption of water in the kidney. It is made by the hypothalamus and secreted by the posterior pituitary gland.

Apgar score   A score out of ten given to newborn babies at one and five minutes after birth. It includes observations of tone, colour, breathing, heart rate and response to stimulation.

BCG   This is 'Bacillus Calmette-Guerin' immunisation, which is an immunisation against tuberculosis.

Body mass index (BMI) (Kg/m2)   The calculation divides an adult's weight in kilograms by their height in metres squared and is used to assess healthy weight, which is a BMI of between 18.5 and 24.99 Kg/m2.

Cervix   Entrance or neck of the womb.

Children's Centre   Children's Centres were created to provide a single place for five key services (early education, childcare, health, family support and help into work).

Chorionic villus sampling (CVS)   A procedure which uses a fine needle to remove some cells from the placenta. It is usually performed via the maternal abdomen although it can be done through the cervix. The fetal cells are then tested for a range of conditions.

Clinical Research Facility (CRF) A specific environment where research staff are housed and patients attend when involved in clinical research.

Colostrum First milk produced during pregnancy and first 2–3 days after birth. Rich in bioactive factors to enhance immunity and promote growth.

Common Assessment Framework (CAF) A standardised approach to assessing the support needs of a parent which is shared across health and social care agencies.

Consanguinity 'Of common blood', when parents are from the same ancestry; for example, when cousins marry.

Corpus luteum Formed in the ovary after release of the egg. It is maintained in early pregnancy and secretes oestrogen and progesterone.

Cotyledons Distinct structures of the placenta (approx. 15–25 cotyledons per placenta) which transmit fetal blood and enable oxygen exchange with maternal blood.

Craniotomy A surgical procedure where a hole is made in the skull. Used historically during obstructed labour to reduce the size of the fetal head and deliver a dead baby.

Crown–rump length (CRL) Measurement made from the baby's head to bottom to estimate gestational age. This measurement is made during ultrasound examination in the first trimester.

Down's syndrome A congenital condition (trisomy 21) where affected babies have an extra chromosome 21 in their cells. Affected babies have distinctive physical characteristics, many have heart defects and all have a degree of learning disability. However, most children with Down's syndrome go to mainstream schools and have a good quality of semi-independent life.

Early Pregnancy Assessment Unit (EPAU) A specialist department where women who experience problems in early pregnancy can attend for diagnosis and treatment. This care includes access to ultrasound scanning where a threatened miscarriage is suspected.

Edwards' syndrome A congenital condition (trisomy 18) where affected babies have an extra chromosome 18 in their cells. It affects many organs, causes learning disability and only 13 per cent of affected babies live past one year of age.

Electronic fetal monitoring (EFM)   Use of an external transducer to detect the fetal heart through the maternal abdomen. This is recorded via a cardiotocograph monitor (CTG) and recorded on paper or digitally.

Embryo   Product of conception from first mitotic division after fertilisation to eight weeks of development.

Epidemiology   The study of the incidence, causative factors and distribution of aspects of health or health behaviour in particular populations.

Episiotomy   A surgical cut made in the skin and muscle of the perineum to widen the opening and facilitate the birth of the baby.

Evidence-based practice (EBP)   When care is based on and informed by the best available evidence.

Expected date of delivery (EDD)   Also known as 'expected due date' and 'expected date of birth'. It is calculated to be 280 days after the first day of the last menstrual period (LMP). Ultrasound scanning in the first trimester will provide a more accurate date.

External cephalic version (ECV)   Manually turning a breech baby into a head-first presentation. Undertaken by a skilled practitioner under scan surveillance.

External os   The opening of the cervix that protrudes into the vagina.

Family nurse partnership (FNP)   A licensed programme of trained family nurses (health visitors or midwives with additional training in the UK) providing support for pregnant teenagers and first-time parents under 24 years of age.

Feedback inhibitor of lactation (FIL)   A protein in human milk that slows milk production when the breast is full.

Fetus   The developing baby from 8 weeks gestation to birth.

4-week quit   Four weeks of abstinence from cigarette smoking which is carbon monoxide verified.

Glycated haemoglobin (HbA1c)   Formed when glucose binds to haemoglobin in the red blood cells, HbA1c levels provide a measure of the level of glucose that has been in the blood in the preceding 2–3 months.

Good Clinical Practice (GCP) training   A requirement for those involved in clinical research and includes instruction regarding keeping research records, taking informed consent and safety reporting requirements.

Gravid Pregnant.

Haemolytic disease of the fetus and newborn (HDFN) A condition where a woman whose blood group is rhesus negative develops antibodies that destroy fetal red blood cells. This can be prevented if the mother receives prophylactic anti-D injections during pregnancy.

Healthy Start A scheme that provides free vouchers for eligible pregnant and breastfeeding women and children under four, to spend on fresh food, milk and vitamins.

Health visitor A registered nurse/midwife who has undertaken additional training in public health. The focus of this role is on monitoring that the baby meets its developmental milestones and addressing any of the issues, such as depression in the mother, safeguarding concerns, etc., that might impede this.

Hepatitis A viral infection affecting the liver, leading to acute and chronic ill health and increased risk of liver cancer.

Human chorionic gonadotrophin (hCG) Hormone produced by the placenta which prevents the ovaries from releasing more eggs. It also stimulates the ovaries to produce oestrogen and progesterone throughout pregnancy.

Human development index (HDI) A measure of average achievement in key dimensions of human development: a long and healthy life, being knowledgeable and having a decent standard of living. Countries are categorised into low, middle and high HDIs. Used as a category in the *Lancet* series on midwifery.

Human immunodeficiency virus (HIV) This blood-borne infection weakens the immune system. Maternal treatment in pregnancy can reduce the risk of transmission to the baby to less than 1 in 200.

Huntington's disease (HD) A degenerative brain disease that leads to changes in cognition, movement and behaviour. If a parent has the disease, there is a 50 per cent chance of the child having the disease.

Induction of labour (IOL) An obstetric intervention to artificially start labour for clinical reasons, such as prolonged gestation or fetal growth restriction.

Infant Describes a child up to the age of one.

Introitus An entrance into an opening, such as the vagina.

Invitro fertilisation (IVF) Where fertilisation of the egg takes place in a petri dish in an assisted conception laboratory.

Lower segment caesarean section (LSCS) The lower segment of the uterus develops at about 28–30 weeks of pregnancy. It has a lower smooth muscle content than the main body of the uterus and is less vascular.

Manual removal of placenta When the placenta does not separate for the uterine wall and needs to be digitally removed by an obstetrician usually in theatre under epidural or spinal anaesthetic.

Maternity Voice Partnership (MVP) An independent group of maternity service users, midwives, commissioners and doctors to review services in light of local need.

Microbiome The genetic material of the communities of bacteria, viruses and fungi that live on and in the body.

Myometrium The muscle layer of the uterus.

National Health Service (NHS) Created by the Minister for Health Aneurin Bevan in 1948, it is the publicly funded healthcare provision for all UK citizens, which is free at the point of access. Services include maternity, general practitioner, hospital and emergency care.

Neonatal During the first 28 days of life.

Neonatal death A liveborn baby (born at 20^{+0} weeks gestational age or later, or with a birthweight of 400 g or more where an accurate estimate of gestation is not available), who died before 28 completed days after birth.

Oxytocin A hormone produced in the hypothalamus and secreted by the posterior lobe of the pituitary gland. It causes contraction of the uterus and ejection of milk. Known as the love hormone, it promotes feelings of bonding, protection and well-being.

Parity How many times someone has given birth.

Patau's syndrome A congenital condition (trisomy 13) where affected babies have an extra chromosome 13 in their cells. It affects many organs, causes learning disability and only 11 per cent of babies live past one year of age.

Patient and Public Involvement (PPI) Involving members of the public in the design and delivery of relevant, ethical and patient-friendly research.

Perinatal mental health   Maternal mental health during pregnancy and for up to one year after the birth of a woman's baby.

Pica   Craving in pregnancy for non-nutritious elements such as coal and chalk.

Posterior pituitary gland   The back of the pituitary gland in the brain that secretes the hormones oxytocin and anti-diuretic hormone (ADH).

Postnatal care   Professional care provided to meet the needs of women and their babies up to 6–8 weeks after birth.

Postnatal period (puerperium)   From expulsion of the placenta to six weeks after the birth.

Pre-implantation genetic diagnosis (PGD)   Following stimulated egg production, eggs are removed and fertilised to create embryos in the laboratory. After a few days, cells are removed and tested for the genetic condition and up to two unaffected embryos are replaced in the womb.

Principal Investigator (PI)   The person responsible for the leadership and conduct of a research study at a local site.

Ptyalism   Increased salivation, sometimes experienced in pregnancy.

Puerperal fever   Bacterial infection of the uterus and/or reproductive tract following childbirth, miscarriage or termination of pregnancy.

Quickening   The first fetal movements felt by the mother.

Random Blood Sugar (RBS)   A blood test taken at any time of day that measures the level of glucose in the blood.

Randomised controlled trials (RCTs)   Research where participants are randomly assigned to receive an intervention or standard care, to find out if the intervention makes a difference to a clinical outcome.

Royal College of Midwives (RCM)   A trade union and professional organisation providing workplace advice and support and online resources to midwives.

Sickle cell disease (SCD)   A serious inherited blood disorder affecting the oxygen-carrying capacity of the blood, associated with painful attacks, anaemia and infection.

Skin-to-skin contact   Where the baby is held in close contact with its mother immediately after birth and until the first feed. It can also be undertaken at other times and fathers also enjoy this closeness.

Spontaneous rupture of membranes When the membrane containing the waters around the baby break naturally and release the amniotic fluid.

Stillbirth A baby delivered at or after 24^{+0} weeks gestational age showing no signs of life, irrespective of when the death occurred.

Surrogacy An agreement, not enforceable by UK law, whereby a woman bears a child for another person. She will be the legal parent at birth, until a parental order or adoption is approved.

Syphilis Sexually transmitted infection which can lead to serious health problems in the baby, or miscarriage or stillbirth. Effective treatment with penicillin can prevent congenital syphilis.

Teratogenic An agent that can cause harm to the developing fetus, such as vitamin A.

Thalassaemia major A serious inherited blood disorder affecting the oxygen-carrying capacity of the blood requiring blood transfusions every 3–5 weeks, injections and specialist care throughout life.

Third-degree tear A tear that happens during vaginal birth, which involves the mother's perineal skin, vaginal wall and muscles around the anus.

Twilight Sleep In the early twentieth century, the two drugs morphine and scopolamine were used during childbirth to produce 'Twilight Sleep' or *Dammerschlaf*. Women would have no memory of the birth.

Urinary tract infection (UTI) An infection in any part of the urinary system; bladder, kidneys, ureters and urethra.

Uterus Also known as the 'womb', the female reproductive organ where the baby grows and develops.

Video Interaction Guidance (VIG) A relationship-based intervention which uses video and feedback to parents to enhance attunement and empathy. Specialist health visitors and child and adolescent mental health workers are the key professionals using this technique.

APPENDIX 1

The PINK study (Baston 2006)

This study used a combined methods approach to follow a cohort of women who had taken part in a prospective survey of their intrapartum care in 2000, known as 'Greater Expectations' (Green et al. 2003). It surveyed women from eight maternity units; four in the north and four in the south of England. That study had used three questionnaires (two antenatal and one postnatal) and women who had completed all three were included in the PINK study.

The PINK study examined how antenatal expectations, intrapartum and postnatal experiences impact on the short- and long-term health of women who have an emergency caesarean birth. To explore the differences in perceptions between modes of birth, all women, irrespective of the type of birth they had, were sent a PINK questionnaire and 738 were returned. Subsequently, 21 women who had an emergency caesarean birth took part in in-depth interviews four years after the birth of their millennium baby.

Analysis of the interview data revealed three interrelated themes: perceived competence, engagement with women and demeanour, and each contributes to a sense of trust in the staff, or lack of it. The core category was identified and named 'intelligent guardianship'. Figure 7.2 (Baston 2006:165) provides diagrammatic representation of how the themes were developed and how the core category 'intelligent guardianship' was developed.

The 'intelligent' aspect of the core category refers to the ability of staff to act intelligently and also to gather and use intelligence (information) to personalise care. Women were most likely to describe staff positively when staff used both their emotional and professional intelligence to assess their well-being. Thus, they had the ability to apply clinical knowledge to the woman's unique situation and work with competence to maintain her trust. Staff also engaged with the woman to identify her individual hopes and fears for the birth; care that involved the woman as a 'key player' was perceived more favourably.

The term that captured the essence of the relationship which women aspired to was 'guardianship' whereby another, appropriately equipped, person took responsibility for their welfare. As 'guardians', the staff acted in the woman's best interest and were there for her when she needed them. Staff had a duty of care and this was shown by their actions. A guardian is not someone you expect will let you down.

Midwives carried out the majority of intrapartum care, but *intelligent guardianship* could be demonstrated by all members of the team, irrespective of whether they had previously met the woman or how long they had cared for her. This was demonstrated by staff who protected women from the urgency of the situation whilst conveying what needed to be done; as a guardian would endeavour to do. When women did not experience *intelligent guardianship* they became vulnerable and experienced negative emotions; for example, when women were left alone during labour they were more likely to become fearful. However, those staff who exercised *intelligent guardianship* enabled women to form an enduring positive experience of birth despite the need for emergency caesarean.

REFERENCES

Baston H (2006). Women's experience of emergency caesarean birth. PhD thesis. University of York, http://etheses.whiterose.ac.uk/14082/.

Green J, Baston H, Easton S, et al. (2003). Inter-relationships between women's expectations and experiences of decision making, continuity, choice and control in labour, and psychological outcomes: Implications for maternity service policy. 'Greater Expectations'. Summary report, Mother and Infant Research Unit, University of Leeds.

INDEX

Printed in the United States
by Baker & Taylor Publisher Services